Introduction

High-protein diets * **Low-fat** diets *
All-vegetable diets * **No-carb** diets *
Hollywood Diets * **Vegan** Diets

...... with all the dieting choices available how do you figure out which one is right for you?

The Lose Weight For Good Diet Bible aims to demystify and explain some of the most popular (and less well known) diet options; offering 101 ideas to help you make the right choice for weight loss success and giving you a roadmap to choose a diet which could work best for you.

The diets are all listed alphabetically (although some are known by a number of pseudonyms which we have attempted to include in the titles). Each diet is then detailed within a series of three key sections along with an additional recommended reading source if you decide the diet might suit your needs and you want to investigate further.

- **What Is It?**
- **How Does It Work?**
- **Who Is It Good For?**

When choosing a diet it's helpful to identify why you want to change or alter your eating habits in the first place. People diet for many reasons; it may be that you are at an unhealthy weight and need to pay closer attention to your eating and exercise behaviours. You could be serial a yo-yo dieter who has tried many fad diets and now want to make a lifestyle change.

Some people may just be looking to improve on their physical condition or have environmental concerns about the food they

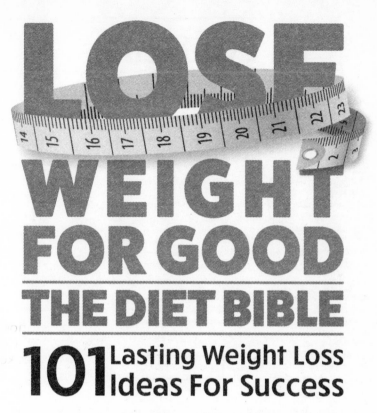

LOSE WEIGHT FOR GOOD

THE DIET BIBLE

101 Lasting Weight Loss Ideas For Success

ISBN 978-1-912155-70-5

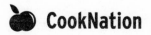

CookNation

Contents

eat, or it could be a new diet is required to help tackle underlying health issues which a poor or unsuitable diet may be contributing to.

The Lose Weight For Good Diet Bible offers you a plethora of possibilities; from the extreme Inedia Diet to a simple Smoothie Diet you should be able to identify a new eating pattern which suits you and your way of life.

None of the diets in this book are in any way endorsed or recommended by CookNation. Whilst every effort has been made to ensure accuracy, descriptions of diets contained in this book may vary from those displayed elsewhere. This book is in no way intended to be an exhaustive resource on the subject of diets and weight loss.

The author and publisher shall have no liability or responsibility to any person or entity regarding any loss or damage incurred, or alleged to have incurred, directly or indirectly, by the information contained in this book

It is highly recommended that you seek the advice of a health care professional before embarking on any diet plan.

About CookNation
CookNation is the leading publisher of innovative and practical recipe books for the modern, health conscious cook.

CookNation titles bring together delicious, easy and practical recipes with their unique no-nonsense approach - making cooking for diets and healthy eating fast, simple and fun.

With a range of #1 best-selling titles - from the innovative 'Skinny' calorie-counted series, to the 5:2 Diet Recipes collection - CookNation recipe books prove that 'Diet' can still mean 'Delicious'!

To browse all CookNation's recipe books visit:
www.bellmackenzie.com

2-Day Diet

What is it?

The 2-Day Diet is an intermittent diet low in carbohydrates that claims to help you become slim and healthy without having to count calories, fast or skip meals. It is claimed that this diet, in addition to weight loss, has numerous health benefits including reducing your risk of cancer, reducing high blood pressure, improving mood and increasing your overall energy levels. This diet is extremely similar to the 5:2 Diet and similar on/off fasting diets.

How Does It Work?

The 2-Day plan is a 5:2 Diet that involves following a low carb meal plan for two days a week and eating normally, within healthy eating guidelines, for the rest of the week. Generally, three meals are to be eaten on low carb restricted days consisting of vegetables, fruits, proteins and a few slow releasing carbohydrates, with the recipes being designed to meet your nutritional requirements and reduce your appetite without increasing your calorie intake. The remaining 5 non-restrictive days are based around a healthy Mediterranean-style diet, which includes whole and unprocessed foods such as plenty of fruit and vegetables, whole grains, low-fat dairy, beans, fish, nuts and olive oil, and limits your intake of red meat, processed sugars and unhealthy fats. The plan attempts to provide clear and simple guidance with nutritionally balanced meal plans and numerous recipes that are designed to help you lose weight without leaving you feeling hungry. The diet also recommends that you drink plenty of water and exercise regularly in order to speed up weight loss.

Who Is It For?

The 2-Day Diet is targeted at those who have attempted various diets and still failed to lose weight, or gained it all back. Additionally, numerous recipes are provided that can be followed by individuals with dietary requirements and preferences.

★ **Find out More:**
The 2-Day Diet
By Michelle Harvie & Tony Howell

Great for....
quick & easy results

3 Hour Diet

What is it?

The Three-Hour Diet recommends that you eat little and often. By eating every three hours you are likely to have six meals a day. Whilst skipping meals is common when dieting, it is believed that this is actually a bad habit to start as this does not help you to lose weight – in fact it can slow down your metabolism.

How Does It Work?

Eating regularly keeps your metabolism going. Where other diets aim to send your body into a state of ketosis, this diet tried to speed it up and maintain a high metabolic rate. This is a much more sustainable approach as ketosis is essentially starvation mode, which cannot be sustained without serious effects in the long term. There is flexibility, so for example you do not need to eat exactly every three hours – sometimes it may be every two hours, other times four – allowing you to tailor it around your typical day.

It is not quite as simple as eating whatever you like six times a day; each time you eat is divided into snack or meal times and you need to aim to keep each 'meal' to around 400 calories, each 'snack' to around 100 calories and each 'dessert' to around 50 calories. Whilst there is a low calorie intake, eating regularly often should help suppress hunger and cravings. Example meal plans are available from author Jorge Cruise which are not too restrictive in nature and do not try to completely eliminate any food groups. You must continue to drink lots of water though, although it is expected that you could lose 10 pounds in a month.

Who Is It For?

The Three-Hour Diet is ideal for those who snack a lot and are often hungry. It is great for a busy lifestyle and if you love your food, as it allows you to still eat a great variety, just in smaller portions. The diet is not targeted at specific groups of people or medical conditions, suggesting it is suitable for almost anyone, however as with all diets, it is recommended that you consult with your GP first.

Great for....
fast results

★ Find out More:
The 3-Hour Diet
By Jorge Cruise

5:2 Diet
The Fast Diet

What is it?

The 5:2 diet is currently the most popular type of intermittent fasting diet.

It was popularized by British doctor and journalist Michael Mosley.

The name 5:2 refers to the seven day week in which 5 days of the week are normal eating days, while the other two days are restricted to eating only 500 calories per day. Although recently this has been revised to 800 calories.

How Does It Work?

You choose which two days you fast on and which 5 days of the week are 'normal days'. On fasting days, you are allowed to drink as many calorie-free drinks as you like. Also you can eat whatever you wish provided it doesn't exceed 500 calories, although healthy & filling low GI foods are recommended as these help you feel fuller for longer. The other 5 days are normal eating days.

Who Is It For?

This diet is great for people who have got busy lives and changing schedules as you can pick your 'fast' days and can therefore be flexible with your eating patterns. Many people find it easier to stick to the 5:2 diet than a continuously controlled calorie restriction. Studies have shown that the 5:2 diet causes weight loss similar to regular calorie restriction and is effective at reducing insulin levels, decreasing inflammation and improving blood lipids.

★ **Find out More:**
The Fast Diet
By Dr Michael Mosley
The Skinny 5:2 Fast Diet
Meals For One
By CookNation

Great for....
flexibility & fast results

7-Day Detox

What is it?

The 7 day detox is a week long program that claims to detoxify your body, increase your natural resistance to illness and encourage your brain to produce feel-good chemicals. This is not a diet for life and it is recommended that the detox should only be carried out 3 or 4 times a year.

How Does It Work?

The 7 day detox is a low-fat, low-calorie diet designed to ensure rapid weight loss. The detox involves a strict and carefully controlled regime, which is high in fruit and vegetables which will flood your body with vitamins and minerals.

The detox varies your calorie intake and what you can eat daily, with Day 1 consisting of a 600 calorie intake of fruit and live natural yoghurt. Also, included in the plan on various days are foods including: fruit juice, vegetables, beans and lentils, tofu, brown rice, fresh fish and herbal teas. Additionally, it is recommended that you drink plenty of water, take additional nutritional supplements to compensate for any vitamin shortfalls, exercise three times a week with a brisk 20 minute walk, and drink healthy juices throughout the detox.

Who Is It For?

The 7 day detox appears to be suitable for everyone and is aimed at those wanting to detoxify their body, cleanse their system and lose weight. The plan is also suitable for vegetarians as it mainly involves vegetables and any meat options can be substituted. However, it is recommended that you follow the plan when you don't have a busy week as you can get headaches when detoxing, also it is advised to consult with your GP before starting a detox.

Great for....
cleansing your body

★ **Find out More:**
7-Day Detox Miracle
By Peter Bennett & Stephen Barrie

The 8-Hour Diet
Time Restricted Feeding

What is it?

Another take on intermittent fasting, The 8 Hour Diet is based on the theory that the human body is designed for periods of eating followed by periods of fasting.

The diet's title refers to a 24 hour day and involves consuming calories over an 8-hour period only and then fasting for a 16-hour period each day.

How Does It Work?

The dieter chooses when they would like their 8 hour eating period to begin. All calories for the day must be consumed during this period only. During the 16-hour fasting period, the human body should be focused on repair and rest, rather than continually digesting food.

There are no forbidden foods on this diet (except sugary drinks) but this is not an excuse to overeat. Portion size must still be a consideration.

You should begin by doing the 8 hour diet three times a week with the idea being you build up to 7 days a week.

Who Is It For?

This diet is great for people who want to lose weight but don't want to deny themselves the things they like. If you are happy to pair this diet with exercise you should see long term lasting results.

★ **Find out More:**
The 8-Hour Diet
By David Zinczenko

Great for....
lasting results

8-Week Blood Sugar Diet (BSD)

What is it?

The 8-Week Blood Sugar is another diet incarnation from Dr Michael Mosley (who developed the Fast Diet). It is multi-stage program that initially involves an intensive fasting plan and then further diet plans which are based around a Mediterranean diet that is low in carbohydrates and places importance on being active. The diet is claimed to aid weight loss and reset your metabolism, with the main aim being to help you lose enough weight to regain control over your blood sugar levels.

How Does It Work?

This diet plan begins with an intensive stage that should be followed for 8-weeks in total. It includes avoiding refined sugar, starchy carbohydrates, and encourages consumption of plenty of vegetables, protein, and moderate amounts of healthy fats that keep you full for longer. Following this intensive stage, you can move onto the more flexible 5:2 BSD, which involves two fasting days on 800 calories and five days on a low carb Mediterranean style diet. Once your weight loss target has been achieved it is recommended that you follow the BSD 'Way of Life', where you stick to a low carbohydrate, Mediterranean diet to sustain your current lifestyle and weight.

Who Is It For?

The Blood Sugar Diet is not targeted for one specific group of people, however as with all detoxes or fasts, these are not always suitable for you if you have some medical conditions. The 8-week fast requires serious willpower and determination, with careful planning and food preparation being required. It is advised to consult with your GP before starting this diet, particularly due to its fasting nature.

Great for....
reducing blood sugar & fast results

★ **Find out More:**
The 8-Week Blood Sugar Diet
By Michael Mosley
The Skinny Blood Sugar Diet Recipe Boo
By CookNation

The 10-Day Detox Diet

What is it?

The 10-day Detox Diet, a low glycaemic and low carbohydrate diet, is based on the idea that the secret to losing weight, and keeping it off, is by maintaining low insulin levels in your body. The diet involves a 10-day meal plan that claims to reduce insulin levels, which aids in losing belly fat, resetting your metabolism, reducing inflammation, and improving your digestive system.

How Does It Work?

The Detox Diet plan is described in detail so that over the 10-days you do not have to make any decisions about what to eat. The plan is designed to make sure you get the correct balance of detoxifying foods and nutrients to reduce insulin levels. The diet involves eating whole, unprocessed foods, mainly consisting of proteins, fresh vegetables, and healthy fats, with all forms of sugar, gluten, dairy, alcohol and caffeine being eliminated. As part of the diet you also get to enjoy a 30-minute UltraDetox bath of lavender oil, Epsom salts and baking soda which is intended to relieve stress. Other recommendations include exercising daily and the use of nutritional supplements. Following the Detox Diet, there are three different plans you can follow, all incorporating the basic principles of the diet with varying degrees of flexibility. Overall, the plan claims to help you lose weight rapidly and followers will learn a healthy lifestyle for prevention of disease and general well-being.

Who Is It For?

This diet is accessible for the majority of people. It is an easy program to follow for a short period of time offering additional guidelines for vegetarians and vegans. The diet claims to correct blood sugar and blood insulin levels, however it is advised you consult with GP beforehand, in particular if you are taking prescribed medication as it may be necessary to monitor your response and adjust doses accordingly.

★ **Find out More:**

The Blood Sugar Solution 10-Day Detox Diet
By Mark Hyman

Great for....

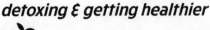
detoxing & getting healthier

48-Hour Miracle Diet
The Hollywood 48-Hr Miracle Diet

What is it?

This diet is designed to achieve rapid weight loss. The diet dictates that you must drink a specifically designed juice every four hours up to four times a day, eat nothing else and drink nothing else aside from water. It is similar to the Liquid Diet in concept; however only the specialist juice mixed with water can be consumed.

How Does It Work?

The juice is mixed with water and is extremely low in calories – only 100 per serving. The low calorie intake, as with many other diets, sends your system into ketosis and your body begins burning its own fat. Through only consuming liquid, the juice moves through your system quicker as well which aids digestion.

It is an intensive diet plan, hence its duration is only 48 hours, however it is said to have incredible results claiming that some participants lose up to 10lb. This diet works like a fast, or as commonly referred to in the dieting world, a 'detox', which indicates that it is not sustainable in the long term and a variety of nutrients are absent.

Who Is It For?

This diet is for the very self-disciplined! It is extremely restrictive and you may be left feeling very hungry. This diet has an extremely low calorie intake and a variety of side effects can be suffered because of this; therefore it is not suitable for everyone, especially for those at a higher risk of hypoglycaemia. Anybody wishing to undertake this diet should consult with a medical professional first, particularly if you have any current medical conditions or take any medication.

Great for....
rapid effects

★ Find out More:
48-Hour Miracle Diet
hollywooddiet.com

Acai Berry Diet

What is it?

The acai berry is not a specific diet plan or schedule as such, but is widely recognised and referred to as a 'superfood'. The acai berry is claimed to have many qualities and health benefits, such as stimulating weight loss and reducing aging. Acai berries are rich in antioxidants and form the base of many diet powders and meal or snack supplements for other diet plans.

How Does It Work?

The concept is that acai berries act as a substitute or enhancement to a meal or snack. Researchers suggest that the acai berry contains more antioxidants than other berries such as blackberries, raspberries and blueberries. It is claimed to aid your immune system, reduce cholesterol and some heart conditions.

Adding acai berries to meals or eating them as snacks, can contribute to a healthy diet through choosing natural foods rather than other processed snacks, chocolate or crisps for example, which in turn can help with weight loss.

Who Is It For?

Acai berries can be eaten by anybody and make a great addition to any breakfast, dessert or snack. As a popular 'superfood', acai berries are often favoured by those who follow diet plans like Clean Eating and Lean in 15 which tend to include superfoods and garner a lot of public attention.

There is some suggestion that if you suffer with pollen allergies, that you should be cautious in consuming a lot of acai, and likewise if you have allergies to other rich berries, such as blackberries, blueberries or raspberries.

★ Find out More:

The Acai Berry Supplement: Alternative Medicine for a Healthy Body
By William Wagner M.D

Great for....
superfood snackers

Alkaline Diet
The Alkaline Ash Diet or Acid-Alkaline Diet

What is it?

The Alkaline Diet essentially looks to replace acidic foods, or 'acid-forming' foods, with alkaline foods. There are a multitude of claims behind this diet ranging from overall health improvement and weight loss, to helping fight cancer. This diet is perceived as more of a lifestyle change and general energy and health boost, rather than a quick-fix weight loss diet.

How Does It Work?

The Alkaline Diet works on the concept that you can change the pH level of your body by controlling the alkaline and acid levels through what you eat. It is explained that once your body has consumed food there is either an acidic, neutral or alkaline effect. A neutral affect is considered to be no problem at all, an acidic effect is perceived as potentially negative, and alkaline has a positive effect. There is some relatively complex science behind this and the theory itself is still argued by researchers.

The belief is that by consuming an alkaline influenced diet, you will see overall health improvements, and potentially even weight loss, however, there are suggestions that it is the consumption of the foods that are typically alkaline, and the reduction of foods that are typically acidic, that leads to the health benefits and weight loss, rather than it being much to do with the acidity or alkalinity itself.

Who Is It For?

Anybody can undertake the Alkaline Diet, although avid meat-eaters may struggle with the significant reduction in meat, poultry and fish. This diet has been popular amongst sufferers of cancer, arthritis and diabetes. Many 'acidic' foods are required however in a balanced diet, so, as with the majority of diets, it is recommended that you seek advice from a medical professional before reducing and/or increasing foods from your diet.

Great for....
boosting energy

★ **Find out More:**
The Alkaline Cure
By Stefan Domenig

Allen Carr Diet

What is it?

The Allen Carr diet was developed by best-selling British author Allen Carr who is best known for his books about smoking addiction, alcohol addiction and other psychological dependencies.

The diet claims that you can eat as much of your 'favourite' foods as you want, whenever you want, as often as you want, and still be the exact weight you want to be, without dieting, special exercise, using willpower or feeling deprived.

How Does It Work?

This diet is more about re-training the mind than almost any other diet on the market. Allen attempts to 'undo the brainwashing' we receive in our modern world which has dictated & distorted what we view as our 'favourite' foods. He suggests our favourite foods are actually those which nature intended for us: ie fruit, nuts and vegetables, rather than the processed foods we are forced into eating.

As such the diet moves you towards getting your brain to believe that following a raw food, vegan plan is both nutritious & healthy as well as being desirable.

Who Is It For?

This diet is good for anyone who wants to understand how modern society has affected our relationship with food. It requires commitment and openness to changing thought patterns. Results for those who embrace the diet are long-lasting and sustainable.

Great for....
*rethinking your
relationship with food*

★ **Find out More:**
Easyweigh to Lose Weight
By Allen Carr

Alternate Day Fasting

What is it?

Alternate day fasting is a type of intermittent fasting.
On alternate days you go between eating normally on one day to eating a very restricted amount of calories the next day. The following day is back to normal eating

How Does It Work?

Day 1 of the diet is a fast day. This means restricting your intake to 500 calories. On fasting days, you are allowed to drink as many calorie-free drinks as you like. Also you can eat whatever you wish provided it doesn't exceed 500 calories, although healthy & filling low GI foods are recommended as these help you feel fuller for longer. Day 2 is a normal eating day. Day 3 is a fast day etc.

Who Is It For?

It's a great way to kick start a diet. Weight loss results can be dramatic provided you don't overeat on your 'normal' eating days.
It can be tough to stick to in the long term but can give great short term results which you can build on with lifestyle changes. It's thought alternate day fasting can also help lower your risk of heart disease and type 2 diabetes.

Great for....
fast & dramatic results

★ Find out More:
The Alternate Day Diet
By Donald R. Laub Sr. MD

Atkins Diet

What is it?

Developed by Dr. Robert C Atkins the Atkins diet is a 4-phase plan which begins by significantly reducing your intake of carbohydrates. It is one of the earliest diet plans using low carbohydrate intake as the underpinning concept and made a big impact following its release in the 70s.

How Does It Work?

Carbohydrates act as one of the main sources of your body's fuel; by reducing your intake of carbohydrates, your body starts to burn its own fat to use as fuel instead, which should result in weight loss. Atkins claimed that in addition to fat loss, you will also experience a number of other benefits such as better sleep patterns, high energy levels, and the reduction of food cravings.

Carbohydrates retain water, and so by reducing them from your diet, you may also lose excess water weight. Atkins, like many other diets, provide a wide range of recipes to suit low-carb meals as inspiration.

Who Is It For?

The Atkins diet appears to be suitable for anyone, however some people do initially experience headaches and feel more lethargic and tired than normal. This is due to retaining less water, and so you can feel more dehydrated. It is clearly highlighted that this diet is not suitable for you if you are pregnant or breastfeeding. There is also a list of medications on their website that if you are taking one or more of, you should also consult with your doctor before starting the diet.

★ **Find out More:**
  The Atkins Plan
  By Dr. Robert C. Atkins

Great for....
reducing that
bloated feeling

Autoimmune Protocol (AIP)

What is it?

The Autoimmune Protocol diet, also known as the Paleo Autoimmune Protocol and commonly referred to as 'AIP', is a stricter version of the Paleo diet concept. It claims to help heal the immune system and gut mucosa (membrane lining) by reducing the inflammation in the gut that causes Autoimmune Disease. This diet aims to flood the body with nutrients to support healing whilst avoiding any food that may be contributing to the disease.

How Does It Work?

Autoimmune Disease is a degenerative condition and is not curable, however this protocol aims to eliminate foods which are triggers for inflammation, thereby calming the gut and immune system and putting the disease into remission. In general, food can be viewed as either promoting health, such as those high in nutrients, or undermining health, such as inflammatory compounds. The AIP emphasises increasing your intake of nutrient-dense foods that promote health and avoiding foods that may trigger your disease.

The plan suggests eating a balanced diet consisting of organic meat, fish and shellfish, vegetables, healthy fats, fruits and fermented foods. The foods to be avoided include: grains, legumes, dairy, processed sugars, oils, nuts, seeds and alcohol. After three to four weeks, if you have seen improvements in your health, you can begin to reintroduce foods into your diet with the recommendation being an introduction of one food every five to seven days and monitoring yourself for symptoms. The protocol claims to work by addressing four key areas that are said to be important contributors to autoimmune diseases, including nutrient density, gut health, hormone regulation and immune system regulation.

Who Is It For?

The AIP claims to be appropriate for everyone with a diagnosed, or suspected, autoimmune disorder. However, it is strongly advised to consult with your GP or specialist before starting this diet especially if you are using it instead of any treatments or if you are taking medication. It is a very strict elimination diet that requires careful planning and patience, so many people may find it difficult to follow.

Great for....

your immune system

★ **Find out More:**
The Autoimmune Paleo Cookbook
By Mickey Trescott

Baby Food Diet

What is it?

The Baby Food Diet is quite simply a diet where you only eat baby food, i.e. small jars or sachets of food that are generally designed for and targeted at babies from the point of weaning. This diet is great for fast weight loss. The Baby Food Diet is popular because of its incredibly low calorie intake (roughly 25 – 75 calories per jar).

How Does It Work?

By eating a jar or sachet per meal, your portion is dramatically reduced and calorie intake controlled. As most food is either puréed or heavily blended, there is little work for you to do in terms of chewing and digesting, and so it is claimed that the food passes through you quicker than usual.

Designed to suit the diets of developing digestion systems of babies, the ingredients are generally quite simple with vegetables or fruits as the staple of each 'meal'. However, because baby food is designed for babies, some food groups are minimised or eliminated completely as is recommended by health guidelines for children under the age of 12 months; therefore, this diet is not necessarily nutritionally balanced for an adult.

Who Is It For?

The Baby Food Diet is great if you struggle to manage portion size as it is already done for you. It is also great for flexibility as there is no fixed rule about how many you can or cannot consume per day. This diet is especially good if you are vegetarian or vegan as many items are a combination purely of vegetables or fruits and often do not contain animal products such as milk or eggs. It is also very quick and easy as no cooking or preparation is required, however eating baby food all day may not suit everyone's tastes..

★ **Find out More:**
The Baby Food Diet
webmd.com

Great for....
Convenient food with no prep

Blood Type Diet

What is it?

The Blood Type Diet is a personalised diet system that is dependent on your individual blood type – O, A, B, or AB. The plan is based on the idea that your blood type is a key genetic factor that impacts on your health and well being, and knowing your blood type is essential in understanding how your body reacts to food, disease, and stress.

How Does It Work?

The Blood Type Diet is based on the idea that, instead of a one size fits all diet, your nutritional needs are determined by your type of blood and that you need to eat the foods that work best for your blood type, allowing you to lose weight, decrease inflammation, increase energy and generally lead a healthier life. It is claimed that the foods you eat react chemically with your blood type, and if you eat the right food your body will digest it more efficiently, producing the beneficial health effects.

It is recommended that those with Type O blood consume a high protein diet, such as lean meat, poultry and vegetables, and limit their intake of grains, beans and dairy. Those with blood type A should consume a meat-free diet based on fruit, vegetables, beans and whole grain, as they have sensitive immune systems. Those with blood type B should avoid wheat, tomatoes, peanuts and chicken, whilst eating green vegetables, eggs and low-fat dairy is encouraged. Those with blood type AB should consume, tofu, seafood, dairy and green vegetables, avoiding caffeine, alcohol and cured meats, as they tend to have a low level of stomach acid. Additionally, the diet recommends exercise based on your blood type, for example gentle exercise for type A's, such as yoga or tai chi, and more vigorous exercise for type O's, such as jogging or biking.

Who Is It For?

The Blood Type Diet is suitable for everyone, with meal plans and advice being available for all blood types. However, the diet requires a high level of effort as you will need to be sure what your blood type is, and depending on your type, you may need to severely restrict what you eat. There is little allowance for specific dietary requirements or preferences, and as always, a medical professional should be consulted before undertaking any diet plan.

Great for....
personalised nutrition

★ **Find out More:**
Eat Right 4 Your Type
By **Peter J. D'Adamo**

Body Building Diet

What is it?

The Body Building Diet is a plan for those wishing to gain a muscular physique through strength training. There is not a single program for all; rather meal plans are often goal-specific and tailored to the individual in order to fuel workouts correctly. Generally, the most important aspect is to increase lean muscle mass, without increasing fat, through a proper eating program that takes in to account your goals, the timing of your weight training, and your intake of macronutrients.

How Does It Work?

A Body Building Diet generally suggests eating six times a day to keep your metabolism steady and stimulate the growth of new muscle. It is generally a low carb, high protein diet that includes foods such as rice, whole grains, proteins, fruit and vegetables. Often, the composition of your meals depends on when you workout, for example strategically eating carbs that slowly increase blood sugar either first thing or directly before weight training, and eating a lot of lean protein throughout the day. Also, it is advised to hydrate regularly and consume whey protein or protein shakes every couple of hours between meals to maximise muscle growth and release fat-burning hormones.

Who Is It For?

The Body Building Diet is aimed at those wanting to increase their muscle mass and is not for everyone, nor is it necessarily a weight loss plan. A number of factors need to be considered when looking to undertake this plan and it is not suitable for all. Several body building websites and personal trainers offer a personalised meal plan that can cater to your nutritional needs, lifestyle and body building goals.

★ **Find out More:**

The Bodybuilding Cookbook
By Jason Farley
Bodybuilding Cookbook Ripped Recipes
By CookNation

Great for....
achieving that
muscular physique

Body For Life Diet

What is it?

Body for Life is a twelve-week program which promises to change your mind, body and life. It is an exercise and nutrition plan that combines weight training and aerobic exercise with a careful daily diet consisting of six small meals (rather than 3 larger meals).

How Does It Work?

The diet is 6 days a week with 1 'free' day (when you can eat whatever you want). On your diet days you can have bread, pasta, potatoes, lean meats, fruits, vegetables, and small amounts of certain fats. You must make sure you eat at least two servings of vegetables and drink 10 glasses of water each day.

At every meal, you get a fist-sized serving each of protein and carbs. Overall, the diet breaks down to about 40% to 50% of each, with very little fat. Foods not allowed include bacon, fatty cuts of beef, hot dogs, deep-fried food, sugary food, cookies, cake, candy, white rice, chips, and fizzy drinks. Butter, lard, mayonnaise, coconut oil, and full-fat dairy products are also off-limits.

Who Is It For?

This diet is great for people who are willing to commit to a twelve week program of diet and fitness. It is also designed to increase your strength of mind which should help you in all areas if your life not just weight loss.

The diet comes with both fitness and meal plans and there is quite a lot of food prep involved.

Great if....
you're time rich and want lasting results

★ **Find out More:**
Body For Life
By Bill Phillips

Body Plan Plus

What is it?

The Body Plan Plus is a 90-day food and exercise journal that is tailored to your calorie needs. This program is not calorie restrictive and claims to be rewarding and sustainable, helping you to lose weight and become healthier.

You also keep a food journal alongside your plan.

How Does It Work?

The Body Plan Plus journal contains several methods that can be used to get you to your goal weight. The plan allows to you to decide how much weight you want to lose and how quickly you want to lose it. Primarily it involves tracking your 'calories in' against your 'calories out', with sections to create a calorie library of the foods you eat which can be used to make a meal plan that fits in with your desired body goals. Generally, it allows you to eat the foods you love in moderation and balance this with calories burnt.

Additionally, the plan contains an exercise system known as the "3 in a row routine", which is designed to be suitable for everyone regardless of your previous exercise history and lets you choose the exercises that are right for your body. This journal has a 90-day food diary so that you can plan, prepare and monitor your progress in a simple way that should only take a couple of minutes each day. Overall the Body Plus Plan encourages you not to change the foods you enjoy, but instead simply become more organised and take control of your diet.

Who Is It For?

The Body Plan Plus is suitable for all shapes and sizes, drawing on the idea that it is suitable for anybody; it allows you to keep eating the foods you love and exercise at a level that suits you best. This plan contains several methods and ideas to help you to achieve your weight loss goal and would suit those who like a well-structured weight loss plan. It is also applicable for those with dietary requirements or restrictions as you can add in the foods you want to.

★ Find out More:

The Body Plan Plus
By Jonathan Bowers

Great if....
*you want to keep
a diary of your progress*

Body Reset Diet

What is it?

The Body Reset Diet is a 15-day plan, consisting of three 5-day phases that aim to increase your metabolism, reboot your system and set your body up for sustainable weight loss in the long-term. It is a low calorie plant based diet that involves initially drinking only smoothies before gradually reintroducing solid foods.

How Does It Work?

The Body Reset Diet has three phases each lasting 5 days. The first phase involves only drinking smoothies for meals, these are packed with fibre, whole grains and vegetables to keep you satiated with each smoothie being colour coded; white is for breakfast, red for lunch and green for dinner. Also, two snacks of around 150 calories are permitted in between meals. The next two phases involve the gradual reintroduction of solid foods into your diet, the second phase replaces one smoothie with a solid meal and the third phase replaces the remaining smoothies with a solid meal. These meals typically are either a salad, sandwich, or stir-fry and are said to all aid in the continuing of weight loss. It is also suggested that you should walk around 10,000 steps a day, which can be done with small lifestyle changes, and the diet should be combined with resistance exercise three times a week.

Who Is It For?

The Body Reset Diet does not target a specific group of people and is a good option for vegetarians This diet may be hard to follow as drinking mostly smoothies is difficult and requires serious willpower and planning.

Great for....
rebooting your system

★ **Find out More:**
The Body Reset Diet
By Harley Pasternik

Bone Broth Diet

What is it?

The bone broth diet is a three-week program that promotes rapid weight loss and elevates the health of your body. It involves a bone broth fast twice a week and the eating of three meals a day for the rest of the week with the meals being in accordance with those recommended. The weekly plan should be repeated twice more for optimal weight loss.

How Does It Work?

Bone broth is said to have several benefits which facilitate weight loss. It gets rid of hunger and the temptation that accompanies it. Additionally, it aids the elimination of toxins from the body, restores your digestive system and reduces inflammation of the body, which can cause weight gain. For the five days each week where food is allowed, restrictive Paleo diet rules are implemented. The overall goal of the diet plan is to place an individual's body into ketosis where fat is burnt for energy instead of carbohydrates, leading to rapid weight loss.

Additionally, if at any point during the three weeks any of the dietary restrictions are not followed within the diet, the diet is restarted to day one. Upon finishing the diet, tips are provided on what you should do in order to not regain the lost weight.

Who Is It For?

The Bone Broth diet is suitable for the majority of people; however as bone broth is made from the meat and bones of animals there is no vegetarian option in this plan and vegetable broth does not provide the same health benefits that contribute to weight loss.

★ **Find out More:**
Bone Broth Diet
By Dr. Kellyann Petrucci

Great for....
fastweight loss

Bulletproof Diet

What is it?

The Bulletproof Diet is a plan which is high in saturated fat, based around a daily cup of coffee with 'upgraded Octane oil' mixed in, which claims to kickstart your metabolism and result in weight loss. This is rather similar in concept to the Metabolism Diet. The diet claims that it will make you feel stronger and leaner, in addition to 'upgrading' your brain and reducing your risks of cancer, heart disease and Alzheimer's disease.

How Does It Work?

The Bulletproof Diet is based on a caloric intake that roughly is made up of 55% from health fats, 20% from animal protein, 15% from vegetables and 10% from carbohydrates.

The program involves consuming a 'Bulletproof coffee' for breakfast, which is made from branded 'upgraded' coffee beans and a spoonful of the diet's own Octane oil – a variant of coconut oil containing triglycerides. For lunch and dinner, it is recommended to eat meals that are high in fat with lots of protein and green vegetables. On the plan, snacking is discouraged and it is recommended that you eat both of your meals within a 7-hour window so your body can fast for the rest of the day, which helps you burn fat faster.

The Bulletproof diet claims to help you lose weight as a high fat and low carb diet places your body in ketosis, the metabolic state where the body gets its energy from fat stores, resulting in your fat being continuously burnt for fuel. This can fuel fast weight loss, however ketosis is a temporary state, and its effects cannot be sustained in the long term as weight loss will begin to stagnate.

Who Is It For?

The Bulletproof diet appears suitable for the majority of people and does not specifically target one group. It is a fairly restrictive plan and may be difficult for some to follow, additionally it is not suitable for some dietary requirements as a lot of red meat is consumed. This diet is not for anyone who is pregnant or breast feeding and it is advised to consult with your GP before starting.

Great for....
coffee lovers

★ **Find out More:**
The Bulletproof Diet
By Dave Asprey

Clean & Lean

What is it?

The Clean and Lean diet is a 14-day meal plan which advocates eating in moderation and helps you change your eating habits through gaining an understanding of what you eat and how it impacts on your body. This is a lifestyle plan that focuses on the key principles of eating healthily and losing weight.

How Does It Work?

The Clean and Lean diet states that the key to weight loss and maintaining a healthy weight is eating light lean proteins and foods that are simply cooked, unprocessed and as close to the way nature made them as possible. The plan claims that by removing 'toxins' from your diet, such as processed foods and sugars, and by focusing on the right foods this keeps your body in the best condition - clean and lean. Clean foods are those closest to their natural state and should be included in a balanced diet along with: lean protein, healthy fats and vegetables. The plan encourages you to eliminate any alcohol, caffeine, 'bad' carbohydrates (pasta and bread) and all sugar, including natural forms. However, one 'cheat day' a week is allowed where you can eat anything you like in order to boost your metabolism and aid in fat burn and weight loss. Generally, being clean means that your body is able to effectively deal with toxins and flush them out, this is essential as it is claimed that toxins cause fat storage, slow down your metabolism and make you feel depressed and tired.

Who Is It For?

The Clean and Lean diet appears achievable for everybody and allows a fair amount of freedom with over 100 recipes to follow and dietary requirements being catered for.

★ **Find out More:**
Clean & Lean Diet
By James Duigan

Great for....
eliminating
toxins

The Clever Guts Diet
The Gut Diet

What is it?

The Clever Guts Diet is another diet offering from Dr. Mosley (who popularised the 5:2 FAST diet). Widely embraced as a groundbreaking concept, Dr. Mosley reveals how junk food and overuse of antibiotics have wiped out much of the good gut bacteria we need. This in turn has led to allergies, food intolerances, and obesity. Drawing on scientific research the diet provides proven ways to control food cravings, boost mood and lose weight by encouraging a more diverse microbiome and increasing the good bacteria that is in your gut.

How Does It Work?

In its simplest terms the diet works by encouraging you to eat the real unprocessed foods that have been shown to encourage the growth of the 'good' bacteria in the gut whilst banning the foods which promote the bad bacteria. This helps cut sugar cravings, boost your immune system and as a result, lose weight naturally. Foods which the diet encourages include fresh seasonal vegetables, fresh seasonal fruit, fresh herbs and spices, unsweetened almond milk, and fermented foods. Things to be avoided include processed/refined foods, alcohol, coffee, soft drinks, hydrogenated fats & gluten.

Who Is It For?

This diet for anyone who want to take a scientific approach to understanding their digestive system and how it affects health. The diet promises to 'revolutionise your body from the inside out' with weight loss not being the goal but often a happy side effect of good gut eating.

★ **Find out More:**
Happy Healthy Gut
By Jennifer Browne
The 28 Day Gut Health Plan
By Jacqueline Whitehart
The gut make over recipe book
By Jeannette Hyde

Great for....
anyone with good gut instincts

The Cookie Diet
The Hollywood Cookie Diet and Smart For Life Cookie Diet

What is it?

The basic premise of Cookie diets is that you eat cookies instead of meals. Of course it's not just any cookie you are allowed to eat. The cookies that are the basis of these diets have been specially made for each of the plans. Cookies are eaten instead of breakfast, lunch, and snacks. Dinner is then of your own choosing but must be 'sensible' or calorie restricted.

How Does It Work?

Cookie diets are simply restricting your calorie intake by swapping regular meals for cookies. Most overweight people are hungry because of insulin and leptin resistance as well as a loss of the hunger control process. The cookies are designed to flip the sugar to protein ratio decreasing sugar and insulin as well as leptin resistance providing the correct protein to sugar ratio.

Eating multiple small meals (cookies)throughout the day delivers specific amounts of protein, fibre, and complex carbs to suppress hunger, whilst keeping sugar and insulin low and triggering the body's fat releasing hormone.

Who Is It For?

This diet is great for people who want simple food options and don't have the time, or inclination, to prepare diet meals. Eating cookies also means you don't feel you are denying yourself treats so it's great if you have a sweet tooth. Results can be very good but for some people eating cookies all day everyday can become boring.

★ **Find out More:**
The Cookie Diet
smartforlife.com

Great if....
you are time poor
with a sweet tooth

DASH Diet

What is it?

The DASH diet is a plan that not only aids with weight loss, but also lowers blood pressure. In fact, it was originally created for the purpose of lowering blood pressure. It is a 14-day plan that has been created as a result of research commissioned by the US National Institute of Health. The DASH diet predominantly focuses on vegetables, fruits, pulses, lentils, wholegrains and foods that are high in protein, but low in fat. Whilst results are expected to be seen fairly quickly, the DASH diet is designed to be maintainable in the long term.

How Does It Work?

The DASH diet plan involves eating a high protein diet that is rich in lean meats, fish and fiber whilst being low in fat. Specific guidelines are provided outlining the number of servings for each category of food you can eat per day. Foods are divided into the following categories: grains and grain products; predominantly wholegrains, fruits, vegetables, low-fat dairy products, lean meat, fish & poultry, nuts, seeds and legumes;. The number of portions are spread across a week allowing flexibility in how you choose to consume them. The balance of the ratio and types of food help contribute to weight loss as well as reducing blood pressure and cholesterol.

Who Is It For?

The DASH diet is said to be suitable for everyone. It is especially good if you have high blood pressure or cholesterol and are looking to reduce both of these issues. An alternative plan is available for vegetarians to suit your diet and maintain the required intake.

Great for....
losing weight & improving your overall health

★ Find out More:
The DASH Diet Plan
By Marla Heller, MS, RD

The Day Diet
The One-Day Super Diet and The 24-Hour Diet

What is it?

This diet goes by a number of names and there are various incarnations. Basically it involves eating strictly for one day of the week; similar in concept but almost the opposite of the 5:2 Diet. Rather than having one or two 'cheat days', you just have one 'diet day', which is perceived to be much more achievable.

How Does It Work?

Your one diet day is lower in calorie intake and restricted to a selection of different foods and meals. Recipes are provided and alternatives included for those who would prefer to buy a ready meal or eat out, making it very convenient. Whilst there is flexibility in the meal choice provided, you must watch and count the calories as per the guidelines, although no specific foods are avoided or eliminated.

Weight loss is achieved as your body is likely to burn more calories than you eat on that one day and you may find that one day of conscious and healthy eating does have a knock on effect on the rest of your week, improving your eating habits as a whole. The non-restrictive nature and small amount of commitment required (one day!) makes this easy to stick to.

Who Is It For?

The Day Diet is ideal for those who get bored easily, struggle to stick to a strict diet plan for more than a few days and if you are looking for a long-term, sustainable fix. As no food groups are eliminated and there is no detox or extreme phase to this diet, it is suitable for anyone - especially those who are busy, constantly on the go and like to eat out.

Great for....
limited
commitment

★ **Find out More:**
The 1-Day Diet
By Jennifer Jolan

The Dopamine Diet
The Tom Kerridge Diet

What is it?

The Dopamine diet is designed to aid weight loss and boost mood by increasing the levels of dopamine in the brain. Often referred to as the 'happy hormone' dopamine has an incredibly important effect on our overall feeling of well-being. Certain foods can help boost dopamine levels and as such focusing on eating these foods is what the Dopamine Diet centers its efforts on.

How Does It Work?

Dopamine affects the reward and pleasure centres in our brains, so the idea is by eating the right type of dopamine boosting foods you not only lose weight but you get happy whilst you do it.

On the diet you are told to eat foods such as eggs, milk, cheese and yogurt, unprocessed meats such as beef, chicken & turkey and omega-3 rich fish such as salmon and mackerel. Also on the hit list are vegetables, fruits, nuts and dark chocolate. Foods which are banned include starchy carbohydrates, processed sugar, alcohol & caffeine. By removing these banned items in favour of healthier protein, fresh fruit and veg options the diet should help you happily lose weight.

Who Is It For?

The Dopamine Diet suits those who suffer from low moods and get 'down' particularly when they are trying to lose weight. There are lots of good recipe options on this diet and as such weight loss can be long lasting and sustainable.

Great for....
anyone who wants to be happy

★ Find out More:
The Dopamine Diet
By Tom Ketteridge

Dukan Diet

What is it?

The Dukan Diet is a 4-phase plan split into two key sections; first, where you lose weight; and second, where you maintain the weight loss. The diet consists of eating from a selected list of foods in each section, and is typically high in protein.

How Does It Work?

The Dukan Diet offers a list of 100 foods; 72 of these can only be eaten during the first part of the plan that covers two phases, the remaining 28 can be introduced in the second part within the final two phases. The idea is that provided you stick to the foods on the list, you can eat as much of them as you like on the allocated days. Your days are split into 'natural protein' and 'protein and vegetable' days and are alternated throughout the week.
Alongside this, an exercise schedule is also provided in all four phases.

Who Is It For?

The Dukan Diet provides personalised plans that are suitable for anyone. The Dukan Diet is not suitable for breastfeeding women and if you are on any medication, it is recommended to consult your doctor first. The diet is either suitable for, or can be adjusted for, various dietary conditions. Results can be long-lasting.

★ **Find out More:**
The Dukan Diet
By Dr Pierre Dukan

Great for....
keeping a wide variety of foods in your diet

Eat-Clean Diet

What is it?

The Eat-Clean Diet is often referred to as the diet that is not actually a diet. It is more a lifestyle regime and attitude to food. The concept of 'eating clean' is to only eat whole foods that are nutritious and responsibly sourced, as well as preparing fresh meals from scratch. Weight loss effects can be seen reasonably quickly and are considered to be long lasting if you adopt this new way of eating.

How Does It Work?

The Eat-Clean diet focuses on eating and cooking with wholesome and natural foods that are not processed and do not have any artificial additives or sugars. Processed and refined sugars are eliminated from your diet, however natural ones are embraced. You are encouraged to eat smaller meals more frequently, so you are often eating throughout the day. It is noted as important to not skip meals in order to maintain your metabolism. Portion sizes can be controlled; however there are few restrictions on what you can eat, although all refined foods should be avoided.

Who Is It For?

The Eat-Clean Diet is suitable for anybody. This diet is good for you if you are looking to make permanent changes to your eating, cooking and shopping habits, and maintain them in the long-term. The Eat-Clean diet is ideal if you struggle to wait between meals as eating smaller portions more frequently can help keep hunger at bay.

Great for....
long lasting effects

★ Find out More:
The Eat-Clean Diet
By Tosca Reno

Eco Atkins

What is it?

The Eco Atkins diet is the vegetarian version of the original Atkins Diet, which is heavily based on non-animal products and provides a meatless low carbohydrate approach to weight loss. The "eco" origin is derived from the diets status as earth friendly. The diet claims to have several benefits in addition to weight loss such as improving cholesterol, controlling blood pressure, increasing energy and reducing cravings.

How Does It Work?

The Eco Atkins Diet maintains the high protein, low carbohydrate and fat-rich approach which the Atkins Diet is originally based on. The meal plan includes protein-rich plant foods along with healthy quality oils and fats that are derived from plant sources. It encourages you to avoid starchy carbohydrates such as rice, bread and potatoes. Generally, the vegetarian version encourages you to skip the first phase of the Atkins Diet and follow the subsequent three stages. The Eco Atkins plan allows 26% of your calories to be from complex carbs such as fruit, vegetables and whole grains. 31% is from plant proteins such as legumes, soy and nuts and the remaining 43% coming from healthy fats such as vegetable oils, avocado and nuts.

By reducing your intake of carbohydrates it is claimed that this causes your body to burn its own fat for fuel resulting in weight loss. Additionally, it is recommended to take a daily multivitamin and flax oil supplement to ensure all of your daily vitamin needs are met.

Who Is It For?

The Eco-Atkins Diet is targeted at vegans and vegetarians enabling them to reap the benefits of the original Atkins Diet whilst fulfilling their dietary preferences. Also, as the diet claims to decrease you cholesterol and blood pressure, it has been suggested as a treatment for heart disease however it is strongly advised that you consult with your GP before following this diet. Additionally it is clearly highlighted that if you are pregnant, breastfeeding or taking some medications, then this diet is not for you.

★ **Find out More:**
Eco-Atkins Diet
By R.M. Lewis

Great for....
vegetarians

Fast Metabolism

What is it?

The Fast Metabolism Diet is a 28-day plan that claims to boost your metabolism and nurture your body back to health without calorie counting by using the strategic targeting of nutrients during a three-phased cycle. This plan is based on the idea that food is not an enemy, but instead is the medicine and fuel that our body needs to revitalise our sluggish metabolism and become fat-burning machines for rapid weight loss.

How Does It Work?

The Fast Metabolism Diet involves eating healthy whole foods as part of a cycle that rotates between rest, rebuilding and burn phases. The first phase takes place on Monday and Tuesday and involves eating lots of carbohydrates and fruits, with these nutrients being used to help unwind stress in the body, allowing you to rest and recuperate.

The second phase takes place on Wednesday and Thursday and involves eating lots of protein and vegetables. This rebuilding phase is designed to unlock fat stored in your body and help build muscle through stimulating less fat storing hormones and more fat releasing ones. The third phase takes place for the rest of the week and involves eating all of the above foods, in addition to healthy fats and oils. This 'burn' phase is said to unleash your metabolism, keeping your stress levels low and fat burn high, while providing you with more energy and a feeling of well being. These phases should then be repeated three more times, with it being claimed that by keeping your metabolism guessing you will get it to work faster and burn more fat, especially from fat stored in problem areas.

Who Is It For?

The Fast Metabolism is targeted at individuals who feel that their sluggish metabolism is getting in the way of their weight loss goals. This program also has an app that provides customised meal plans, food lists and numerous recipes, including organic, vegetarian, and gluten-free options.

Great for....
a metabolic energy boost

★ **Find out More:**
The Fast Metabolism Diet
By Haylie Pomroy

Fit for Life

What is it?

The Fit for Life Diet is a lifestyle program based around food combination theories that focus on weight loss occurring due to the eating of 'correct' food groups and avoiding 'wrong' combinations. The idea is this provides stable weight loss and can maintain effects in the long term.

How Does It Work?

It is suggested that certain combinations of foods, known as 'dead foods', can clog the body and these foods include meats and starches. The foods that cleanse the body are known as "living foods" and these include raw vegetables and fruit. The Fit for Life plan requires that these foods cannot be eaten together. Additional rules include: fruits are healthy only if they are eaten in isolation and not in combination with other foods; proteins and carbohydrates should not be eaten together; dairy products should not be eaten; and water should not be drunk at mealtimes. However, the individual can have one free day a week that allows them to eat whatever they want to.

This lifestyle plan aims to teach individuals to be healthier. Weight loss should occur, not through exercise or counting calories, but through avoiding eating foods rich in carbohydrates and proteins at the same time and allowing enzymes to properly digest each food type separately.

Who Is It For?

The Fit for Life program is claimed to be suitable for individuals of all ages and their personalised diet is intended to be one for a lifetime. However, due to the elimination of dairy products and restrictions on food types, individuals must consult with their GP if they are concerned about vitamin and mineral deficiencies.

★ **Find out More:**
The Fit For Life Diet
By Harvey and Marilyn Diamond

Great for....
a personalised lifetime change to your diet

Five Bite Diet

What is it?

The Five Bite Diet is a low-calorie diet based on the simple principle that if you eat less you will lose weight. The diet involves counting how bites of food you take rather than how many calories you consume. This diet claims that a portion-controlled plan is the most effective strategy for sustainable weight loss and that how you eat is more important than what you eat. Unlike other diets that control portion size, you are not required to measure or weigh anything – you simply stick to five bites. This is great for rapid weight loss.

How Does It Work?

The Five Bite Diet involves you skipping breakfast and then you are allowed only five bites of your food at lunch and dinner. Generally, the plan allows you to consume whatever foods you like as long as you have some protein each day and take a multivitamin supplement, although it is encouraged to stick to a healthy diet that focuses on nutrient-dense foods, such as whole grains, fruits, vegetables, low-fat dairy and lean protein.

It is also encouraged to drink as much as you want as long as you stick to those that are calorie free. Because you are eating only a few bites daily, even if you take large bites and eat high calorie foods, this low cal diet is designed to recalibrate how your body measures feeling 'full' and leads to rapid weight loss. The diet encourages you to stick to this plan until you have reached your goal weight and then you can go back to eating normally.

Five bites, even for those with larger than average mouths, is not very much and so this is similar to a daily fast. The weight loss is therefore unlikely to be sustainable in the long term.

Who Is It For?

The Five Bite Diet is designed for those wanting rapid weight loss results. As this diet is very restrictive and low in calories you'll probably be quite hungry throughout the day so you will need will power. It is advised to consult with you GP before beginning this diet, especially if you are elderly, unwell, pregnant or breastfeeding.

Great for....
rapid weight loss

★ **Find out More:**
Why Weight Around
By Dr. Alwin Lewis

Food Combining Diet

What is it?

Food Combining dieting is based on the idea that certain foods pair well together whilst other foods do not and the diet plan specifies how different food groups should be combined as a meal. The proper combination of foods enhances your digestion and allows you to gain the maximum amount of energy and nutrition from the food you are eating. With an enhanced digestion you can feel more energetic and healthier which encourages a healthy relationship with your weight.

How Does It Work?

There are two ideas behind the rules of food combining. Firstly, the digestion of different foods occurs at different rates and can cause a blockage in your gut leading to negative digestive and health outcomes. Also, these different food groups require different levels of acidity in your digestive tract and if foods are eaten together that require a different level of acidity, then they cannot both be digested properly at the same time.

The food combing diet involves following three main food consumption principles that aid the process of digestion. Firstly, fruit should be eaten alone as they are one of the easiest of foods to digest. Secondly, protein should be paired with non-starchy vegetables as the enzymes secreted to break down protein produce an acidic environment that is not ideal for the breakdown of starchy foods. Thirdly, starches should be eaten with non-starchy vegetables as the enzymes secreted to break down starches produce an alkaline environment - one that is not ideal for the digestion of protein. These principles are the core of the diet; however further principles do provide rules for the food combining of oils, fats and dairy products.

Who Is It For?

The food combining diet should be suitable for all as there are several plans to accommodate different dietary requirements and preferences based on these food-combining principles, with recipes and sample menus being provided.

★ **Find out More:**
The Body Ecology Diet
By Donna Gates

Great for....
more energy &
less digestive distress

Forks Over Knives Plan

What is it?

The Forks Over Knives Plan is a vegan diet that is based on a feature documentary, called "Forks Over Knives", which examines how the Western Diet affects our bodies and is making us sick – similar to the concept of the Mad Diet that advocates the benefits of switching to a plant-based diet. The plan aims to ensure that people stick to a healthy nutritional and well balanced vegan diet and stay away from convenient junk foods.

How Does It Work?

The Forks Over Knives Plan involves consuming whole, unrefined or minimally refined plants and meals generally consisting of vegetables, fruits, tubers, legumes and wholegrain. So quite literally eating foods that only require a fork, not a knife. It is emphasised that these should all be consumed as part of a balanced plan because a diet of mainly vegetables is not sustainable and will not contain the nutrients that your body needs. It is suggested that in addition to vegetables you should eat healthy fats, such as avocados or nuts, and starchy vegetables that bulk out your meals, such as sweet potatoes, brown rice and beans. As the diet is high in fibre this helps you feel fuller for longer. The plan encourages you to eliminate meat, dairy products and eggs in addition to highly refined foods such as white flour, oil and sugar. The diet also provides lifestyle advice and encourages followers to eat mindfully and listen to their body as this can help you know when you are full and stop you from overeating or craving sugary foods.

Who Is It For?

The Forks Over Knives Diet appears to be suitable for everyone. The plan is easy to follow through the use of their recipe app, which is frequently updated with new and seasonal recipes and also allows you to create a shopping list. Some individuals may find this diet difficult at first as it involves eliminating a lot of common foods from your diet

Great for....
a vegan lifestyle

★ **Find out More:**
Forks Over Knives
By Gene Stone

G Plan Diet

What is it?

The G Plan Diet is a three-phase gut-friendly plan that lasts 21-days and claims to improve your overall health and help you reach your weight loss goals. The overall aim of this diet is to eliminate foods that are bad for the bacteria in your gut and replace these foods with gut-friendly ones to soothe and rebalance your digestive system. Additionally, the diet provides followers with information on how the gut microbiome is linked to a reduced risk of illness, improved mood and weight loss along with a practical guide to follow in order to reap the benefits. This diet is not dissimilar to the Louise Parker Method, just with fewer 'phases'.

How Does It Work?

The G Plan Diet has three phases in total. The first phase, known as "Rest" phase lasts 5 days and involves eliminating all processed and junk food from your diet such as foods containing refined carbs and sugar, giving your digestive system a much needed break. The second phase, known as "Re-Wild" phase, lasts 9 days and involves reintroducing gut-healthy pre- and probiotic foods and drinks into your diet, such as kefir, miso, pickles, garlic, bananas and sauerkraut. This phase should leave you feeling more 'with it' and slimmer. The third and final phase, known as "Rebalance" lasts for 7-days and involves the reintroduction of foods that are potentially difficult for your digestive system, allowing you to monitor how you react to different foods. The G Plan Diet encourages a more natural and diverse diet and aims to provide you with new, healthier cooking and eating habits. It is claimed that eating a diet that keeps your gut happy also has an impact on your health: your skin glows, you lose that bloated lethargic feeling and lose weight.

Who Is It For?

The G Plan Diet appeals to those who want to rebalance their digestive systems and lose weight. The plan is easy to follow with lots of batch cooking and freezing of meals in order to fit in with your daily life. This is suitable for those with dietary requirements or preferences as you can swap out the ingredients you don't like for the ones you do.

★ **Find out More:**
  The G Plan Diet
  By Amanda Hamilton

Great for....
soothing your gut

GERD Diet

What is it?

Gastroesophageal Reflux Disease (GERD) occurs when a specific muscle in the lower oesophagus weakens and allows stomach acid to splash up into the oesophagus resulting in various symptoms, including heartburn and chest discomfort as well as fluid flowing directly upwards into the mouth. The GERD Diet was designed in order to prevent, or at least reduce, the amount of acid reflux and aims to ease the symptoms and calm the disease when combined with other lifestyle changes.

How Does It Work?

The GERD diet claims to combat acid reflux and allows followers to consume the basic food groups – cereals, vegetables, fruit, dairy products, and meat – with only a couple of restrictions. Typically, the diet encourages avoiding foods that may aggravate acid reflux such as fatty or fried foods, mint, creamed foods, caffeine, citrus foods and chocolate. The GERD diet varies from person to person and must be tailored uniquely. The plan encourages you to monitor the way your body responds to different foods so that you can devise the best meal plan possible to help you manage this condition.

If you are unable to tolerate citrus foods it is recommended that you take Vitamin C supplements to ensure you get your daily amount of essential vitamins and minerals. Other guidelines include avoiding nicotine as this weakens the lower oesophageal muscle, avoiding late evening snacks and lying down after eating. Eating small, frequent portions of food should make for slow, steady weight loss.

Who Is It For?

This diet is designed specifically for those suffering with GERD although it has been suggested that it may also aid some other common digestive problems. The GERD Diet requires patience, time and planning in order to find the plan that is best for you, however it is not too restrictive and should be easy to follow. It is highly recommended that you consult with you GP before attempting this diet especially if you are currently taking medication for your condition.

Great for....
relieving reflux

★ Find out More:
101 Best Foods To Treat & Cure GERD
By Health Research Staff

Gluten-Free Diet

What is it?

A gluten-free diet is implemented for various medical and dietary conditions (most commonly coeliac disease or gluten intolerance), however it is now popular as part of a weight-loss routine as well. Gluten is found in wheat, barley and rye, therefore any foods or drinks that contain any of these grains (or traces thereof) must be avoided when pursuing a gluten-free diet.

How Does It Work?

Regardless of whether you suffer from coeliac disease or gluten intolerance, eating a gluten-free diet, or at least swapping refined grains for wholegrains, can help with weight loss. This is mainly due to the fact that wholegrains are rich in fibre, which can help reduce bloating and cravings as you feel fuller for longer. Weight loss itself is stimulated more by cutting out foods that typically contain gluten, such as carbohydrates like bread and pasta, rather than stimulated by the absence of gluten, as is commonly misunderstood.

Who Is It For?

For dietary purposes, a gluten-free diet would be implemented for you if you are suffering from coeliac disease, gluten intolerance, IBS or dermatitis herpetiformis, for example. However anybody can choose to undertake a gluten-free diet for weight loss benefit, although it is recommended to consult with your doctor first.

★ **Find out More:**
Gluten-Free Diet For Beginners
By Kira Novac

Great for....
gut intolerance

The Grapefruit Diet

What is it?

The Grapefruit Diet determines that you should eat half a grapefruit before every single meal. There is no one specific dietary plan or program to follow, although grapefruit does play a small role in many diet plans and has a reputation for boosting your metabolism. Some 'Grapefruit Diets' promote diet plans high in protein, whereas others combine it with a limited calorie intake; however the main underlying idea is quite simple.

How Does It Work?

Grapefruit is believed to have many beneficial qualities to our health and unlike some other 'superfoods' that are commonly found in popular diets, there is a fair amount of scientific research to back up grapefruit's benefits.

Grapefruit is one of the healthiest fruits in the citrus family due to its low-calorie, high-nutrient qualities and also contains a large number of vitamins and minerals. It is also an antioxidant and believed to suppress your appetite and reduce cravings. With this in mind, the majority of grapefruit diets provide that you should eat half a grapefruit before each meal. Studies conducted showed that when added to participants' daily diet, the participants went on to lose weight and benefited from a reduced waist size.

These benefits were shown to be just from consuming half a fresh grapefruit before meals. In some of the diet plans available, grapefruit juice is also included in the program or meal plan, however there is an argument that this does not have the same benefit as the fresh, natural fruit.

Who Is It For?

This diet is really suitable for anybody, especially those that want a really easy way to shift some pounds without compromising your current diet; however, whilst this can aid weight loss, do not expect to lose vast amounts of weight by this idea alone.

Great for....
an easy fix

★ **Find out More:**
Benefits of Grapefruit
Healthline.com

Green Smoothie Diet

What is it?

The Green Smoothie Diet is very similar to the Smoothie Diet. The main difference is just that the options for smoothie ingredients are much more limited and there is a large 'clean eating' influence. The Green Smoothie Diet has been incorporated into a number of different detoxes and fast plans, including the 3-Day Green Smoothie Diet, the 10-Day Green Smoothie Diet and the 30-day Fat Burn Diet.

How Does It Work?

There is no specific plan or schedule to follow, other than that some, or in sometimes all, meals are replaced with a smoothie of low-calorie content. Green Smoothies, as expected, consist of predominantly 'green' foods that by nature are typically low in fat and calories. A wide range of vegetables and fruits can be combined and blended to create a Green Smoothie. Typical examples are broccoli or apple and of course the explosion of 'superfoods' has brought spinach, kale and avocado to the forefront of many diets, paving the way for the popularity of Green Smoothies.

This low-calorie, low-fat, liquid diet allows you to lose weight quickly as your body begins to burn its excess fat. However, as with any fast-acting diets where some food groups and products that would usually contribute to a balanced diet are eliminated, this diet is not sustainable in the long term. If solely consuming Green Smoothies, weight loss will reach stagnation. Green Smoothies have however found a market for replacing snacks, breakfast or some drinks to provide an immune system and energy boost.

Who Is It For?

This diet comes in a variety of forms and each form and interpretation thereof, can be suitable for different people. If used as an enhancement to a nutritious diet or replacement of snacks, then green smoothies are suitable for anybody. If looking to undertake a fasting diet where the Green Smoothie is all that you consume, it is highly recommended that you consult with a health professional first.

★ **Find out More:**
The Green Smoothie Recipe Book
By Mendocino Press

Great for....
green leaf lovers

The Harcombe Diet

What is it?

The Harcombe Diet is based on the idea that there are three common conditions; food intolerance, candida and hypoglycaemia, that cause food cravings. These conditions themselves arise from restricting your calories when eating. The diet states that in order to resolve these conditions and lose weight you need to stop counting the calories and eat real food, making the calories that you do eat count, allowing you to lose weight for the long term.

How Does It Work?

The Harcombe Diet involves scrapping fake and low nutrient food and instead eating real food high in nutrients. The program includes three phases in total with recipes and support being provided both in books and online. The first phase lasts for 5 days and allows you to eat an unlimited amount of meat, eggs, fish, natural yoghurt, vegetables (excluding mushrooms and potatoes), and "safe" grains such as brown rice and quinoa. The diet encourages you to eat three meals a day and only eat snacks, such as raw carrot, when hungry.

The second phase lasts for as long as is required for you to reach your goal weight and is based on three main rules: avoid processed foods, don't mix fats and carbohydrates in the same meal and avoid the foods that give you cravings. In this phase you are allowed to reintroduce some more foods including dairy products, fruit, baked potatoes and whole grains. The third phase starts when you are at a weight that you can easily maintain, known as your natural weight, and is meant to last for life. This phase claims to teach you how to 'cheat' while maintaining your weight - generally saying that you can enjoy any food or drink whenever you want as long as you don't cheat too much or too often and always stay in control.

Who Is It For?

The Harcombe Diet appears to be suitable for everyone, in particular those who experience cravings for certain foods or who may suffer from the conditions stated above. However, as with any medical condition you should consult with your GP before starting the Harcombe Diet.

Great for....
banishing cravings

★ Find out More:
The Harcombe Diet
By Zoe Harcombe

The Hay Diet

What is it?

The Hay Diet is a plan based on the idea that the chemical process of digestion affects your health. The diet intends to implement permanent changes to your digestion. The diet classifies foods into acidic, alkaline and neutral groups and provides rules as to how these groups should be combined at meal times. The correct combinations improve digestion, aid weight loss and can treat medical conditions associated with obesity.

How Does It Work?

The diet states that proteins should be eaten at one meal, carbohydrates at another and you should wait for at least four hours between the two incompatible meals. This is because the body uses an alkali process to digest carbohydrates and an acidic process to digest protein, thus if consumed at the same time the acid process interrupts the alkaline ultimately leading to weight gain as energy is drained. Acidic foods are protein rich, such as meat and fish, whereas alkaline foods are carbohydrate rich, such as potatoes and rice. Vegetables are considered neutral and can be consumed with both food groups. Primarily the diet consists of consuming fruit and vegetables as they are low in calories, rich in fibre and give a sense of fullness all of which lead to weight loss. Some versions of the Hay diet place an emphasis on eating small portions of starches, proteins and fats and others place emphasis on avoiding processed foods that contain refined sugar and white flour.

Who Is It For?

The Hay diet is not specifically targeted to one audience although it does state the health benefits for treating medical conditions including constipation, arthritis and heart disease. Importantly, those diagnosed with a medical condition should consult their GP before commencing the Hay diet and may still require medication in addition to a weight loss program.

★ **Find out More:**
Health Via Food
By Hay William

Great for....
relieving medical conditions

High-Protein Diet

What is it?

Opposite to the Low-Protein Diet, the High-Protein Diet states that increasing your protein intake has several beneficial effects on your metabolic rate, appetite, body composition, body weight and general health. It has been stated that for weight loss and overall health approx. 1.2 – 1.6 grams of protein per kilogram should be consumed (making up around 25% of your daily calorie intake) although there is some controversy surrounding the optimal amount of protein to consume for effective weight loss.

How Does It Work?

Protein is an essential nutrient that serves a number of important functions in the body including tissue repair and maintenance and supporting hormonal and enzymatic body systems. Different food types provide better forms of protein than others based on their amino acid composition. Animal products are considered "complete" proteins as they contain all of the essential amino acids that our body needs, whereas vegetable proteins have to be combined with other foods to make them 'complete' proteins. There are a few general guidelines to follow including keeping a food diary, calculating your protein needs, eating well balanced meals and ensuring the protein is from high-quality sources. With some plans also emphasising a low consumption of carbohydrates.

Eating more protein aids the suppression of hunger and appetite, making you feel fuller for longer and leading to a decrease in eating. Overall, through these effects, the high-protein diet is effective for improving body composition and gradual weight loss.

Who Is It For?

The High-Protein diet can be customised for vegetarians and vegans. There are several popular variations of this diet so there are plenty of options if you feel one particular form is not working for you. These diets may cause problems for individuals with certain medical conditions or diseases so you should consult with your GP before undertaking any plan.

Great for....
effective weight loss and overall health

★ Find out More:
High Protein Classics
By Louise Kang

High Residue Diet

What is it?

Residue refers to material that is not digested in the gut or is left from foods containing fibre. The High Residue Diet plan involves eating foods high in fibre as they are involved in digestive health through promoting the movement of food in the gut and give bulk to your stool. It is recommended that 20 to 35 grams of fibre is consumed each day.

How Does It Work?

The High Residue Diet recommends foods high in fibre including cereals, certain fruits and vegetables, legumes and whole grains. The undigested fibre is essential in the maintenance of a healthy bowel and regular bowel movements, as well as playing a role in controlling blood sugar levels and aiding weight loss. The fibre allows you to feel full without majorly increasing your calorie intake, making you less likely to be hungry and therefore encouraging you to eat less.

This is a gradual way to lose weight as fibre must be slowly introduced into your diet otherwise a drastic increase can result in digestive distress and stomach cramping.

Who Is It For?

This diet plan is relatively easy to follow and not overly restrictive. The high residue diet is often prescribed in the treatment of digestive problems including constipation. However, it is important that you consult with your GP before embarking on this diet. Also a high fibre diet may not be ideal for some conditions such as irritable bowel syndrome.

★ **Find out More:**
  High-Fibre Diet Book
  By Dr. Andrew Stanway

Great for....
improving digestive health

Hormone Reset

What is it?

The Hormone Rest Diet is a 21-day plan that claims to reset the efficiency of your major hormones by repairing and growing new receptors for them. The result is an increased metabolism making you lose weight, and helping to reverse the signs of aging. It consists of seven 3-day resets designed to help you get your metabolic hormones back into balance one by one and leave you feeling great.

How Does It Work?

The Hormone Reset Diet focuses on seven major metabolic hormones. The diet claims that when you develop a resistance to these hormones your body adapts by raising your hormone levels and decreasing your metabolic rate. This hormonal imbalance then leads to fat storage and weight gain making it difficult to lose again no matter what you try. The plan lasts 21-days in total and involves 7 resets, one for each major hormone, that occur one at a time each taking 3-days. For example, the first hormone to be reset is oestrogen and tackling the imbalance of this hormone involves avoiding conventionally raised red meat, said to increase oestrogen levels, and instead eating pastured grass-fed beef that helps to repair and restore your metabolism.

The plan provides guidelines as to what you should eliminate depending on which hormone you are resetting at the time. Following the resetting of all of your major hormones you are encouraged to reintroduce foods and separate the foods that you can tolerate from the ones that you can't through monitoring your symptoms. The program also provides advice on how to balance your mental state using a combination of mindfulness and other technique. Advocating the benefits of relaxation and positive emotions on your hormone balance, diet and overall well-being.

Who Is It For?

The Hormone Reset Diet is most suitable for those who feel they may have a hormonal imbalance which is interfering with weight loss. This diet does seem to appeal more to women than men, but is not specific to one hormone. This plan is simple to follow but requires planning and patience for over a month.

Great for....***rebalancing your system***

★ Find out More:
The Hormone Reset Diet
By Sara Gottfried

Inedia Diet
Breatharian Diet

What is it?

The inedia diet is an extreme diet which consists entirely of fresh air and sunlight. Followers of the diet believe that fresh air contains the life force 'prana' and that this, coupled with sunlight, is all that is needed for survival.

How Does It Work?

Food and water are to absent from this diet. The extreme nature of this is an esoteric practice which attracts those who wish to heighten their spirituality through fasting. Believers claim the diet has little to do with losing weight; although some attest to the health benefits and lightness of body that follows an extended period of fasting. Traditionally short periods of fasting have been undertaken for spiritual, religious, political or health reasons however the Inedia Diet is an extreme practice that has been linked to numerous deaths by devout followers who died from dehydration or hypothermia. It has been unanimously rejected by medical and health communities.

Who Is It For?

This diet is for people who wish to have a short term esoteric experience by removing food and water from their life.

Try if ....
you want to have an esoteric experience for a short period of time

★ **Find out More:**
A Year Without Food
By Mr Ray Maor

The Inuit Diet

What is it?

The Inuit diet involves primarily eating foods that are eaten by traditional Inuit people. This includes foods that are hunted, fished for or obtained locally. This diet does not tend to include much plant life as little grows in the freezing temperatures where this diet originated. The majority of food is eaten raw, frozen or boiled, with two meals being consumed each day with frequent snacks. The Inuit people only eat when they are hungry so meals are not set at certain times.

How Does It Work?

The Inuit diet aims to keep the body strong, warm and healthy through the primary consumption of meat and animal blood, such as seal meat and blood when it is still warm. Other hunted foods include walrus and raw or frozen salmon. It has been said that those on this diet rarely feel ill due to this healthy way of life.

This diet is specific to Inuit life and is focused on a cultural way of eating rather than a diet to lose weight.

Who Is It For?

The Inuit diet is limited to certain geographic regions due to the availability of fresh seal, fish and meat, thus very few people can successfully follow this way of life and experience the health benefits.

Bizarre but....
great for boosting your health

★ Find out More:
The Eskimo Diet
By Dr Saynor & Dr Ryan

Jenny Craig Diet

What is it?

Jenny Craig is an American subscription service that delivers food straight to your door with multiple meal options and snacks. The subscription allows a personalised menu and provides individuals with support through neighbourhood weight loss centres and a dedicated personal consultant. The subscription also now incorporates Jenny Craig "Anytime" which provides one to one support on demand either online or on the phone.

How Does It Work?

On this meal plan you eat six times a day, consisting of three meals and three snacks. It is recommended that a wide variety of low calorie and high volume foods are eaten so that you feel fully satisfied. The program allows you to personalise the meals that are sent to you from a wide range of premium options. Weight loss is successful as the program is nutritious, makes eating well easier, provides continual support and weight loss coaching, and creates a pattern of healthy eating that last for a lifetime.

Who Is It For?

Jenny Craig appears to be suitable for anyone. The program allows you to personalise what you eat and can work for vegetarians and for those with other specific dietary requirements. Additionally, as the meals are prepared for you and delivered to your door this is a very convenient program that requires little effort with regard to food preparation.

★ **Find out More:**
Jenny Craig
jennycraig.com

Great for....
convenience and eating a variety of foods

The Juice Fasting Diet
Juice Feasting, Juice Diet, Juice Cleanse or Juice Detox Diet

What is it?

Juice Fasting is a specific period of time when the only thing consumed is liquids; specifically water, herbal teas, fresh fruit and vegetable juices. Solid foods are not consumed at all as the fibre content activates digestion which should be avoided during fasting. The following liquids; coffee, caffeinated teas, milk, fizzy drinks, pasteurised juice, protein powder mixes and diet drinks are also not allowed.

How Does It Work?

When you fast, your body is using all the time normally spent on digestion to clean up (detox) your cells. It's estimated almost three quarters of a person's energy every day is spent on digestion alone, so when you are eating regularly throughout the day you are rarely giving your body a chance to direct energy to cleansing and drawing up acidic waste that may be causing you health problems.

When you juice fruits and vegetables you remove the fibre and drink only the liquid which contains the nutrients, vitamins and enzymes from the plant food. Cutting out regular eating whilst you fast can see some dramatic results and many of the Juicing Diets around make impressive claims of weight loss in as little as a week. There is no doubt that juicing has changed people's lives and for dedicated followers juicing has become a permanent lifestyle choice.

Who Is It For?

This diet is good for anyone who wants to see dramatic weight loss and experience a detox. It requires will power (and a love of fruit & veg).

★ Find out More:
The Juice Master's Ultimate Fast Food:
Discover the Power of Raw Juice
By Jason Vale
The Skinny Juice Diet
By CookNation

Great for....
quick results!

KE Diet
Feeding Tube Diet

What is it?

The KE diet, which is also referred to as the feeding tube diet, is a diet that consists purely of a specific mixture called 'KE diet powder'. The dieter only consumes this powder mixed with water for the duration of the diet, but can drink water as well as sugar and milk-free tea & coffee.

How Does It Work?

The KE diet powder is mixed with water and is all you consume for 10 days. The mixture is fed to you through a tiny feeding tube directly to your stomach;. The mixture contains only proteins, fats and vitamins and they claim that the absence of carbohydrates and sugars will force your body to burn fat. It is believed that the fat burning process is intensified because the mixture is fed straight to your stomach. It is claimed that during this diet, you will lose weight but feel no hunger. Despite being invasive no surgery is required, however medical supervision is necessary.

Who Is It For?

The KE diet does not exclusively target a certain group of people, however they do state that it is not suitable for you if you have had any serious medical or mental health issues. If you wish to do this diet, you must undertake a medical history as well as physical, blood and psychological tests and checks before proceeding.

★ Find out More:
   KE Diet
   By Dr. Oliver Di Pietro

Great for....
quick and easy results without having to do anything

Ketogenic Diet
Keto Diet

What is it?

The Ketogenic Diet is another low-carb diet with a focus on eating whole and natural foods, or 'real' foods as they are commonly referred to. This mainly includes preparing and cooking from scratch rather than eating processed or pre-prepared meals, as well as selecting ingredients based on their sourcing, i.e. grass-fed animals when choosing meats, free-range products etc., in line with a wholesome and ethical approach. Whilst results can be seen quite quickly, the Ketogenic Diet's focus is on adopting a healthier lifestyle and attitude to food for long-term benefits and weight control.

How Does It Work?

The Ketogenic Diet splits foods into a traffic light-like system whereby foods are divided into colours: green – you can eat these foods freely; amber – you can eat these foods occasionally; red – you must avoid these foods completely. You are able to eat any and all meat, albeit grass-fed, healthy fats and non-starchy vegetables; keep fruits, nuts and some vegetables to a minimum; and avoid factory-farmed meats, processed foods, low-fat and low-carb products, alcohol and milk. By not having to process artificial foods, carbohydrates and unnaturally fatty foods, your body begins to process food better and burn fat more effectively.

Who Is It For?

The Ketogenic diet is thought to be suitable for anyone. It is noted that it is particularly good in lowering insulin levels and so can benefit those with diabetes. The diet can be challenging for vegans as there is not a huge range of options that you can freely eat to sustain a balanced diet.

Great for....
a long-term lifestyle change

★ Find out More:
The Keto Diet Cookbook
By Martina Slajerova

Lean in 15

What is it?

Lean in 15 is a book series, developed by personal trainer Joe Wicks (The Body Coach) that contains high nutrient 15-minute meal recipes and high-intensity workouts. The aim of the plan is to end low calorie diets and instead fuel your body with grains and healthy fats that are able to sustain you throughout the day and during a workout thereby keeping you lean and healthy. This is a long-term lifestyle change, rather than a quick fix diet, although results can be dramatic.

How Does It Work?

The Lean in 15 book provides numerous meal and snack recipes that are nutritionally balanced, consisting of healthy carbohydrates, good fats and high levels of protein. The book encourages you to fuel your body with the right food at the right time and take control of your diet using the quick and easy recipes provided. This plan prides itself on being a simple approach that helps burn fat, build lean muscle and makes sure you never go hungry, this paired with high intensity exercise aids you with your weight loss goals.

The Lean in 15 program involves tailoring your meals to your levels of exercise, with three different sections for training days, rest days and snacks. Generally, on a training day when you are planning to exercise, you are advised to eat three meals rich in carbohydrates and two snacks. On a rest day, you are advised to eat three reduced carbohydrate meals and two snacks.

Who Is It For?

The Lean in 15 recipes and workouts are not targeted to a specific group of people and appear suitable for anyone. The book includes a number of easy-to-follow recipes that can be tailored for those with specific dietary requirements and give you the freedom to eat a variety of different foods. This diet is great for food-lovers who enjoy spending time in the kitchen as preparation is key.

★ **Find out More:**

Lean in 15
By Joe Wicks, The Body Coach

Great for....
*getting
(and staying) lean*

Liquid Diet

What is it?

The Liquid Diet involves only consuming liquidised foods. A liquid diet is calorie controlled and can deliver dramatic results very quickly. The longevity of the diet, however, is questionable, and not all of the weight loss may be sustainable in the long-term. You can create a liquid diet yourself by blending and juicing foods, or you can buy products and 'meals' that are already prepared for you.

How Does It Work?

There are few limitations as to what you should and should not include as part of the diet, however for practical reasons, fruit and vegetables are a staple part of the liquid diet. Equally, soups and broths are great alternatives rather than overloading on sweet fruits. There is a wide selection of recipes online and preparation is key. Some liquid diets are solely liquid; others may include a combination where only some meals are replaced with a liquid alternative.

Weight loss is experienced due to the controlled number of calories.

Who Is It For?

Anyone can undertake a liquid diet, and it is highlighted that liquid diets can be especially effective for people who suffer with Crohn's Disease. There are some potential side effects, such as fatigue and dizziness, which may result if essential nutrients are eliminated and so consultation with a doctor is advised before beginning the diet.

Great for....
quick weight loss

★ **Find out More:**
The Liquid Diet
Livestrong.com

Louise Parker Method

What is it?

The Louise Parker Method is a six-week program of sensible healthy eating, daily exercise and positive thinking. The plan claims to be different from all other diets as it is realistic, easy to follow and sustainable. Its concept and regulation of which foods you should and should not eat, is quite similar to many other diets which combine diet, exercise and lifestyle. This 'method' combines elements of 'Clean Eating' and 'Lean in 15' as well as 'Hormone Reset', albeit not to the same extreme.

How Does It Work?

The Louise Parker Method is based around 'Four Pillars" that should be followed completely for six-weeks in order for you to lose fat, maintain a healthy metabolism and feel healthier both mentally and physically. The first pillar, 'Thinking Successfully', involves the challenging of your mind set to previous diet failures and weight loss. The second pillar, "Live Well", involves stress management and sleeping well in order to rebalance the hormones that support weight loss. The third pillar, "Eat Beautifully", involves eating three meals and two snacks a day, all containing unprocessed foods that are a good mix of low-GI carbs, protein, and healthy fats in a portion size that results in a calorie deficit. Additionally, alcohol is banned and you should eat your meals at a table. The fourth pillar, "Work Out Intelligently", involves exercising everyday in a time efficient way without having to rely on a gym; this includes 10,000 steps a day and daily toning workouts. These pillars are all said to help you in your weight loss journey and provide you with a lifestyle change that is healthier and sustainable.

Who Is It For?

The Louise Parker Method seems to appeal to everyone and in particular targets those that have tried other diets and found that they have not worked. There are several meal plans to follow to keep you on track with your weight loss and fitness goals and this plan can fit in with most dietary requirements.

★ **Find out More:**

The Louise Parker Method: Lean for Life
By Louise Parker

Great for....
a sustainable diet

Low-Carb High-Fat Diet

What is it?

There are numerous variations of low carb high fat (LCHF) diets, for example the Atkins or Ketogenic diet, which are said to aid in weight loss through increasing your metabolism and burning of your fat stores. Other health benefits are said to include a decreased risk of heart disease and reduced inflammation.

How Does It Work?

Generally, a LCHF diet involves consuming around 70% of your caloric intake from healthy fats and 30% from proteins, with small amounts of carbohydrates from vegetables, such as leafy greens.

The low-carb component is said to be an effective way to keep your insulin levels low, this is important when you consume a large amount of fat as high insulin levels can lead to the storage of fat in the body. The high fat component is said to encourage your body to burn fat as a primary source of energy, so both the consumed healthy fats and the fat stored in your body are burned, resulting in weight loss and a leaner you. Additionally, protein is said to have appetite-suppressing effects, causing you to eat less, with vegetables high in fibre leaving you feeling fuller for longer. Foods to avoid include refined oils, fruit, alcohol, sugar and starchy carbohydrates, such as wheat, rice and potatoes.

Who Is It For?

LCHF diets seem to be suitable for anyone, with some diets targeting those with insulin resistance or diabetes due to the low carb component. The diet can be tailored to the individual with various meal plans being available to meet your dietary requirements or preferences. However, as with any diet it is advised to consult with your GP before starting.

Great for....
keeping insulin levels low

★ Find out More:
Low Carb High Fat Cookbook
By Sten Sture Skaldeman

Low Fat Diet

What is it?

A low fat diet involves a reduction of saturated fat in your diet; this can aid the reduction of your calorie intake, improve cholesterol levels and promote healthier food choices, ultimately leading to weight loss. High fat foods also tend to have a high content of carbohydrates, so a low fat diet can potentially reduce blood sugar levels as well.

How Does It Work?

A low fat diet should be balanced to include a healthy amount of both vitamins and minerals. Foods included are whole grains, lean meats, white fish, fruit and vegetables, and reduced fat dairy products. As fat has a higher number of calories per gram than either protein or carbohydrates, reducing fat intake should decrease your calorie intake overall and can make you feel fuller for longer, leading to weight loss. This diet also stipulates between the different types of fats, with saturated ones being 'bad' and unsaturated ones being 'good'. The good fats can be found in nuts, oily fish and avocados, and are thought to be largely beneficial for us.

Who Is It For?

This diet is not specifically targeted to one group and appears to be an option for the majority of people. For some medical conditions, such as diabetes, the low fat diet can alter the blood glucose levels and so it is recommended to consult with a medical professional before commencing the diet. This diet requires the careful planning of meals and identifying of 'good' and 'bad' fats, however there are several meal plans and recipes available to follow.

★ **Find out More:**
Low-Fat Low-Cal
By Good Housekeepng Institute

Great for....
long term steady weight change

Low Fod Map

What is it?

The name FODMAP refers to a type of carb known as Fermentable Oligosaccharides, Disaccharides, Monosaccharides & Polyols.
For susceptible people this carb can draw water into the digestive tract and create the uncomfortable sensation of feeling bloated. For must people Fodmaps are not a problem but for others they can aggravate existing health issues.

How Does It Work?

The diet is Gluten free, low sugar and is designed for health benefits rather than weight loss (although weight loss may occur when the diet is followed). It concentrates on removing FODMAPs from your diet and whilst there are many foods you can eat, there is a steep learning curve to figure out which foods are high in FODMAPs and what you should replace them with instead. If you follow the diet closely it's estimated you should start feeling the benefits within about 4 weeks.

Who Is It For?

This diet is great for people who suffer from bloating, belly pain, diarrhoea, constipation, IBS, Crohn's disease, coeliac disease and other digestive disorders.

Great for....
sufferers of digestive problems

★ Find out More:
The Low FODMAP Solution
By Shasta Press

Low GI Diet

What is it?

GI is standard for Glycaemic Index; the low GI diet involves eating foods that have a low score on the glycaemic index (GI), a measure of how quickly carbohydrates are broken down into glucose. Foods with a low score, such as whole grains, nuts, beans and lentils, can stabilise blood sugar levels as they release their energy more slowly. The idea is to keep your blood sugar levels; unsurprisingly the diet was originally designed for those with diabetes.

How Does It Work?

Low-GI foods encourage slow and gentle rises in glucose levels leading to a small increase in the level of insulin, which keeps you feeling fuller for longer and more energised in comparison to high GI foods which produce a sugar rush. Low-GI foods can also speed up the body's metabolism of fat as there is less glucose in the blood to utilise for energy and so fat is burned instead. Also, high-fibre foods are recommended as they take longer to digest and keep you full, leading to a decrease in calorie intake.

Who Is It For?

This diet is targeted for those with diabetes, however it can be followed by almost anybody as it is a great way of making better, healthier food choices and cooking better, healthier meals. There are various meal plans you can follow all based on the GI of foods. Additionally, it has been suggested that this diet is particularly good for individuals wanting to regulate their blood sugar levels and promotes healthier life choices that can last a lifetime.

★ **Find out More:**
Low Glycaemic Diet
By Dr Axe

Great for....
balancing blood sugar

Low GL Diet

What is it?

Glycaemic Load (GL) is a unit of measurement that indicates how a certain food will alter your blood sugar level, with foods that have a higher GL affecting your blood sugar more – an effect which is not desirable. A diet involving Low GL foods, it is claimed, encourages the body to burn fat as they are slow releasing and keep your blood sugar balanced, which results in sustainable weight loss.

How Does It Work?

When your blood level is increased, such as when you eat High GL foods, this causes insulin to be released to breakdown glucose; excess glucose gets turned into fat and stored resulting in weight gain. A Low GL Diet is said to aid weight loss as The Low GL Diet involves two stages; a weight loss stage where you should eat no more than 40GLs daily and a weight maintenance stage in which 65GLs can be eaten. The Low GL Diet provides meal plans and guidance on how foods add up to your daily allowance with various recipes that you can follow.

During the weight loss stage you are allowed to consume three meals (10GLs each), 2 snacks (5GLs each) and a dessert (5GLs), with it being encouraged to eat little and often in order to keep your blood sugar level balanced. Generally, a low GL meal consists of some low GL carbohydrates, such as soy products, beans and whole grains, with plenty of protein as this helps to slow down the release of sugar and does not affect the balance itself. The Low GL Diet also recommends that healthy fats should be eaten and bad ones avoided, you should exercise daily for at least 15 minutes and supplements can be taken to ensure you get all of the essential minerals and vitamins your body needs.

Who Is It For?

The Low GL Diet appears to be suitable for most individuals, in particular those who wish to regulate their blood sugar levels and lose weight. The diet plan is fairly unrestrictive, has various recipe options that can be followed and caters for all dietary requirements. If you are considering following this diet it is advised that you consult with your GP, especially if you are currently taking medication for controlling your blood sugar levels.

Great for....
avoiding sugar 'crashes'

★ Find out More:
The Low-GL Diet Bible
By Patrick Holford

Low Protein Diet

What is it?

The Low-Protein Diet involves reducing your daily protein intake and is often a plan prescribed for those with certain medical conditions including metabolic disorders or kidney and liver diseases. The Low-Protein Diet is quite self-explanatory - a plan to implement changes to your diet to decrease the volume of protein you consume which is, unlike many other diets where the aim is to increase your protein intake..

How Does It Work?

The Low-Protein Diet aims to reduce the workload placed on your kidneys and liver so that the healthy parts do not have to work as hard to digest protein and also prevents the build up of harmful waste products in your blood that result from eating too much protein. The two main sources of protein include animal products, such as meat, fish, eggs and dairy, and vegetable products containing lower amounts of protein, such as breads, cereals and beans. The overall idea is to limit your intake of protein by 'extending' the protein in your meals, for example by eating thinly sliced sandwich meats, soups, and meals mainly consisting of vegetables and grains. By eating a low-protein, lower calorie diet and minimising fats, your body will begin to burn the excess fat it has whilst still maintaining energy levels.

Who Is It For?

This diet is generally suitable for those who need to reduce their protein intake for medical reasons. Dieters should consult with their GP before beginning a Low-Protein Diet and should also consider the natural decrease in calorie intake that is associated with this diet.

★ **Find out More:**
Low Protein Diet
By Robert Galarowicz

Great for....
reducing strain on the kidneys

Low Sodium Diet

What is it?

Sodium is a mineral that is naturally found in foods and is also added to foods, with the primary source being table salt. Due to sodium's essential role in the body's fluid balance and blood pressure, a Low-Sodium Diet is often suggested to aid with cardiac symptoms or disease. The main source of sodium is of course salt, and so this diet looks specifically at reducing your salt intake as much as possible.

How Does It Work?

Due to the role of sodium in maintaining the fluid balance in your body, it is thought that limiting your intake of sodium will control the build up of fluid around vital organs or in your legs. This is because carrying extra fluid makes your heart work harder and can increase blood pressure.

Generally, the guidelines for this diet suggest avoiding using table salt on food and eliminating foods with a high salt content or with added salt, as is often the case with processed convenience foods. It encourages followers to eat fresh, minimally processed foods or low sodium alternatives and read the information on food labels to check how much sodium is present. It is claimed that avoiding excess sodium, can lead to changes in your eating habits, which along with a decrease in excess body fluid can aid weight loss.

There is speculation as to whether the reduction in salt actually aids weight loss or whether weigh loss occurs because foods typically high in salt (takeaways, burgers, ready meals, etc.) are avoided and so calorie intake is decreased.

Who Is It For?

The Low-Sodium Diet does not specifically target a group of people, although there is a particular emphasis on the benefits of this diet for those with high blood pressure or certain heart conditions. If your diet is high in salt, then it is recommended by many health professionals to reduce this. However salt is still a vital element for our bodies, so if your diet is not particularly high in sodium, this plan may not provide many benefits for you. As with all diets it is recommended you consult with your GP before altering your eating patterns.

Great for....
heart health

★ Find out More:
The Easy Low Sodium Diet Plan
By Christopher Lower

Macro Fit

What is it?

The Macro Fit Diet states that it is a flexible approach to dieting which focuses on food composition - the macro-nutrients, micro-nutrients and fibre that make up food. The plan aims to provide a practical diet that is maintainable and produces sustainable results

How Does It Work?

The Macro Fit Diet involves eating foods, including protein, carbohydrates and fats, which meet your daily calorie and macronutrient targets. The plan provides a system that quantifies the composition of foods, allowing you to monitor your daily intake in order to meet your desired goal and maintain good health. The diet places an emphasis on consuming micronutrients and fibre, with around 80% of your daily intake being from whole foods that are minimally processed and nutrient-dense. With 20% coming from any other foods that allow you to reach your daily macronutrient target. This diet produces a unique plan based on your calorific needs, metabolism, and health goals, ensuring you have targets that are the most effective for muscle growth, fat burning and consistent energy levels.

Who Is It For?

The Macro Diet appears to be suitable for anyone and is tailored to your specific needs. It requires some planning and preparation but is easy to follow and fairly unrestrictive. There are several plans that can be followed, providing numerous recipes, fitness advice, and catering for dietary requirements.

★ **Find out More:**
IIFYM: Iff It Fits Your Macros
By Jon Peterson

Great for....
flexibility

Macrobiotic Diet

What is it?

The Macrobiotic Diet is a Japanese-style food plan which includes rules about food and kitchenware. It is based on Zen Buddhism and the balance of yin and yang food elements. The main principles include eating less animal products, more locally grown foods, and avoiding foods containing toxins. The creator of this plan believed that through this diet people could live in harmony with nature and also believed that it could cure cancer and many other diseases.

How Does It Work?

The Macrobiotic Diet is based on 10 plans that can be progressed through in order to reach an ideal ying to yang ratio of 5:1. The foods with yang qualities are considered heavy, hot, dense and compact, whereas ying products are light, cold and airy. Generally, the emphasis is placed on meals eaten in moderation that combine local whole grains, pulses, vegetables, beans, lentils and fermented soy, with wholegrains being consumed the most; as these are considered to be the closest to a ying/yang balance. Due to a further emphasis on avoiding foods containing toxins, many people follow a completely vegan diet.

Unusually, this diet also has guidelines for the use of kitchenware; utensils should be made from only glass or wood and electric ovens should be avoided, with an overall emphasis on preparing your food in a peaceful environment.

Who Is It For?

This diet is suitable for most dietary requirements but it does require careful planning and preparation.

Great for....
developing body and soul

★ Find out More:
The Macrobiotic Way
By Michio Kushi

Mad Diet

What is it?

The Mad Diet takes a different approach to most diets; suggesting that the pressures on people to lose weight are actually having greater impacts on mental health. The Mad Diet looks at losing weight in a sustainable way that is not another 'fad diet'. Suzanne Lockhart, the author, explains how an unhealthy diet could be linked to the increase in mental illness and other health conditions. The 'Western' diet is highlighted as the route cause and definition of an unhealthy diet and the eating plan tries to steer the dieter away from this.

How Does It Work?

This diet is a politically charged piece of food writing that works by opening your eyes, and mind, to the darkly deceptive nature of the food industry. Amongst other things it highlights the scale of artificial additives and sugar which are added to food and the unhealthy manner in which food is both consumed and purchased....aided by the selling techniques of supermarkets and the complicity of government.

Who Is It For?

The Mad Diet targets those who are struggling to lose weight, may have difficulty with mental illness or want to understand the reality of the modern western food industry.

★ **Find out More:**

Mad Diet: Easy Steps to Lose
Weight and Cure Depression
By Suzanne Lockhart

Great for....
peace of mind
weight loss

Magnetic Diet

What is it?

Created by former serial dieter Nick Smith the Magnetic Diet aims to achieve weight loss and enhance overall well being by harnessing the powers of food magnetism.

How Does It Work?

On this diet the foods you eat work with your body to promote a better sense of wellness with their 'magical' properties. The Magnetic Diet teaches you how to deal with your food cravings. Since the main reason people fail on their diet program is because of unplanned food indulgences, if you are able to overcome this, it is a step in the right direction. The diet also explains "the mathematics of weight loss" which is essentially planning out your ratios of carbohydrates, protein and fat along with how they comprise the total calorie intake of your diet. The diet plan takes a very well rounded approach to nutrition and also introduces some meditation practices that allow you to improve the overall quality of your life.

Who Is It For?

This diet is good for someone who is looking to improve their overall meal planning and eating habits. However it requires an 'open mind' with regard to harnessing food's 'magical' magnetic properties.

Great for....
new age thinkers

★ Find out More:
The Magnetic Diet
By Nick Smith

The Master Cleanse
The Lemonade Diet

What is it?

Master Cleanse is a liquid only diet based around a simple lemonade recipe.

The diet consists of 3 basic things; a lemonade-like beverage, salt-water drink, and herbal laxative tea. The diet is an extended detox which can last up to 14 days in its initial period. Benefits of the detox can include weight loss, increased energy, balancing of your Body's pH, allergy relief & improved skin amongst other things.

How Does It Work?

The Master Cleanse lemonade drink is a combination of freshly squeezed lemon juice, organic maple syrup, cayenne pepper and water. After drinking only this for between four and fourteen days solid food is slowly introduced back into the diet, beginning with foods like vegetable soup, followed by fruit and vegetables. Some versions of the diet also recommend a probiotic supplement. People lose weight on the Lemonade Diet because it is more of a fast than a diet, and there are simply very few calories ingested. Its extreme low calorie intake inevitably causes faster weight loss than a more conventional diet.

Who Is It For?

This diet is good for anyone who wants to see fast, dramatic weight loss and experience a detox. It requires significant will power and whilst some people experience a euphoric feeling on the diet others suffer from headaches, fatigue, dizziness, sluggishness, diarrhoea, nausea and constipation.

★ **Find out More:**
The Master Cleanse
By Tom Woloshyn

Great for....
a quick fix

Mediterranean Diet

What is it?

The Mediterranean Diet is considered a heart-healthy eating plan that is based on the typical foods and recipes used in Mediterranean-style cooking which incorporates healthy eating basics, healthy oils and even the occasional glass of red wine.

How Does It Work?

As there are many countries located around the Mediterranean Sea there is no single correct way of following this diet. Generally, most diets include vegetables, fruits, fish, nuts and whole grains, and emphasise replacing unhealthy fats with healthier ones such as olive oil. Other guidelines can include limiting your intake of red meat, regular physical activity, drinking red wine in moderation, and enjoying your meals with friends and family. The Mediterranean Diet does not directly limit the total amount of fat you consume but rather encourages you to make wise decisions about the types of fat you eat, with olive oil being the preferred choice. Overall, the diet appears to be more about promoting healthy lifestyle choices in order to improve health, whilst claiming to reduce the risk of heart disease, other chronic diseases, and lower the levels of 'bad' cholesterol.

Who Is It For?

The Mediterranean Diet provides a general lifestyle guideline and the plan can be adjusted to suit your individual needs, preferences or specific dietary requirements, making it potentially suitable for anyone. Although drinking wine is suggested, this is optional and should be avoided by anyone who may have trouble controlling their alcohol intake or other alcohol related issues.

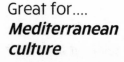

Great for....
Mediterranean culture

★ **Find out More:**
The Everything Mediterranean Diet Book
By Connie Diekman and Sam Sotiropoulos
The Skinny Mediterranean Diet Recipe Book
By CookNation

Modified Fast
Protein Sparing Fast

What is it?

A protein-sparing modified fast is a very low calorie diet that includes vitamin and mineral supplementation. The diet is not a permanent lifestyle solution and is undertaken during a short and specific time period.

How Does It Work?

The idea of the diet is to reduce calories to the lowest possible threshold whilst still eating enough protein to preserve lean tissue mass and enough micronutrients to avoid deficiency.

The diet is very low calorie to try to encourage your body to induce a starvation response (as with all fasting diets). The vast majority of calories should come from lean protein with fat and carb intake being minimal. Supplemental vitamins and minerals need to be taken to make up the inevitable nutrient and electrolyte deficiencies.

Who Is It For?

This diet is good for people who want to kick-start rapid weight loss. It provides fast results which can be very motivating and is useful for someone starting their weight-loss journey. It is particularly suited to very overweight people who want to see results fast. It is however not sustainable over a prolonged time period.

★ **Find out More:**
PSMF Meals
By Maggie Jones

Great for....
heavier people who want to kick start their weight loss fast

Never Binge Again

What is it?

Never Binge Again is a coaching program, designed by a former food-obsessed psychologist. It provides one-to-one help and specific techniques to overcome cravings, lose weight and stick to a food plan of your choice. Unlike many 'fad' diets, this is a long-term plan to change your way of eating permanently for steady and maintainable weight loss.

How Does It Work?

The Never Binge Again program is designed for those who struggle with food, find it difficult to stick with a healthy diet or have gained weight back that they have previously lost. The plan aims to change your mind-set and improve your ability to stick to a healthy food plan so that you can achieve and maintain your weight loss goals. Through the coaching program it is said that you will gain a healthier mind-set and be able to free yourself from the food obsessions that interfere with your maintaining a healthy diet and losing weight. The program involves various techniques and several worksheets including a custom food plan and food plan templates, overcoming binging and challenging your food obsessions. Additionally, one-to-one support is provided both online and through phone calls. Overall, the program does provide some food plans but focuses more on correcting your thinking so that you can follow any healthy diet plan.

Who Is It For?

The Never Binge Again program is designed for individuals who struggle to stick to healthy diets due to their unhealthy food obsessions. The plan involves changing your mind set and because you can chose a diet that suits you, is suitable for any dietary requirements.

Great for....
overcoming food obsessions

★ Find out More:
Never Binge Again
By Glenn Livingston Ph.D.

Nourish & Glow Diet

What is it?

Nourish and Glow is an illustrated guidebook that provides a 10-day meal plan aimed to help you lose weight, change your lifestyle to a healthier one and become confident in knowing what diet works best for your body. The plan is based on the concept of 'Positive Nutrition', which is the opposite to restrictive dieting and involves understanding what we should be eating and what our bodies need us to be eating; this is similar in part to other diets such as 'Clean Eating'.

How Does It Work?

Nourish and Glow claims to be an essential guide for those wishing to live a healthier life, with the 10-day meal plan revolving around the Positive Nutrition Pyramid which is easy-to-follow and promises to change not only the way you eat, but also how you cook and shop for food. The Pyramid, which is implemented in the meal plan, suggests the importance of different food types in your diet. It is encouraged that vegetables should be consumed the most followed by: fresh fruit, protein, complex carbs, healthy fats, and nuts and seeds, respectively. The guide includes a well-balanced meal plan that is said to contain all of the essential nutrients needed for a healthy body and happy mind.

Who Is It For?

The Nourish and Glow guide appears to be suitable for everyone; it is easy to follow, not overly restrictive, only requires some planning and has recipes available for all dietary requirements and preferences.

★ **Find out More:**
Nourish & Glow
By Amelia Freer

Great for....
a healthy glow

Nutrisystem Plan

What is it?

The Nutrisystem Plan is a subscription diet that provides portion-controlled meals and snacks to manage weight loss. By using the right balance of nutrients, Nutrisystem offers specific plans and menus that allow you to start losing weight immediately. They deliver the selected/planned food so all the preparation is done for you and the portion control is out of your hands.

How Does It Work?

Nutrisystem design meals and snacks to include the right mix of nutrients for your body whilst keeping the calories managed. By providing foods that are low in fat, but high in protein and fibre, and controlling the portion sizes, the majority of the work it already done for you. The food you select is delivered to your door and by following the schedule and eating what they send, you can begin losing weight immediately. Nutrisystem also include a fitness plan during the later stages of your 4-week plan.

Who Is It For?

Nutrisystem provide a variety of plans which they say can suit anyone. They have specific plans for vegetarians, males and females and medical conditions, such as diabetes. Many people like the 'ready to eat' nature of this diet and the fact that little preparation is required, as everything is done for you.

Great for....
a busy lifestyle

★ Find out More:
The Nutrisystem Plan
Nutrisystem.com

Paleo Diet
The Caveman Diet

What is it?

The Paleo Diet is a lifestyle diet that involves eating the same foods as our ancestors once did, with followers aiming to eat as naturally as possible. It is believed that our digestive systems have remained the same and that certain foods which have become everyday foods we eat actually put a strain on our gut. The Paleo Diet takes a real back to basics approach and has some similar underlying concepts to the Alkaline Diet.

How Does It Work?

The Paleo Diet includes grass-fed meats, plenty of fruit and vegetables, and wholefoods like nuts and seeds. Dieters are encouraged to avoid dairy-products, potatoes and grains, however some more 'relaxed' variations of this diet do allow these "taboo" foods. Other foods to be avoided include cereals, salt, processed foods, legumes, alcohol, caffeine and refined sugars. Overall, the diet tends to be low in carbohydrates, high in protein, plant foods, fibre and nutrients that keep you feeling fuller for longer. Processed and 'modern' foods are a big 'no-no' but there are no limits to portion size of approved foods.

Additionally, due to the decreased strain on our digestive system and increase in nutrient-dense foods, the Paleo diet is said to have many health benefits, including improved blood sugar control and a reduction in the risk factors for heart diseases. Weight loss follows as a natural consequence of no longer eating processed high calorie foods.

Who Is It For?

The Paleo diet does not target a specific group of people and there are several variations of the diet that can be followed. Some people may find this diet difficult due to its restrictive nature and need for careful planning and preparation. As always, when eliminating any food groups from your diet, it is recommended to consult with a health professional first.

★ **Find out More:**

Paleo for Beginners
By John Chatham
The Paleo Cookbook
By Rockridge Press

Great for....
a back to basics lifestyle

Pioppi Diet

What is it?

The Pioppi Diet is a 21-day lifestyle plan based on a Mediterranean style diet inspired by Pioppi, a small fishing town located in southern Italy. The diet is similar to The Mediterranean Diet, and focuses on avoiding added sugar and carbohydrates, and building a balanced diet around vegetables and natural fats. This plan also includes healthy living advice, incorporating guidelines for exercise, breathing, sleep and spending time with family and friend. The plan claims to change your lifestyle into a healthier one without calorie restriction or endless hours at the gym.

How Does It Work?

The Pioppi Diet encourages you to eat between five and seven portions of vegetables high in fibre and low-fruit sugar per day, with the majority of portions being vegetables. It is also recommended to have a couple of tablespoons of olive oil and a few nuts every day. Other foods that are highlighted include oily fish – around three times a week, eggs, full-fat dairy, dark chocolate, and a small glass of wine. The foods to avoid include all added sugars, refined carbohydrates including bread, pasta and rice, and limiting your intake of red meat. The Pioppi Diet also suggests that each week followers should have one fasting period lasting 24-hours, in order to burn up excess fat and increase your metabolism. This method of eating should produce steady long-term weight loss. The program also includes a movement protocol for the duration of the plan to ensure followers stay active and also includes stress-busting exercise movements and short breathing exercises.

Who Is It For?

The Pioppi Diet provides a general guideline that covers all aspects of a healthy lifestyle. The plan has a number recipes to follow that are relatively easy to prepare and can be tailored to your dietary requirements. Drinking wine is suggested in this plan, however this is optional and should be avoided by anyone with a history of alcohol problems.

Great for....
an Italian twist

★ **Find out More:**
The Pioppi Diet
By Dr. Malhotra and Donal O'Neill

The Primal Diet

What is it?

The Primal Diet is based on "The Primal Blueprint", a plan which allows only foods that our primal ancestors would have had access to; focusing on protein, natural fats, and plenty of vegetables in their most natural state such as organic foods and unpasteurised or raw dairy products. The Primal Diet is considered to be a lifestyle choice and is meant to be sustainable in the long-term. This diet is very similar in many ways to the Paleo diet, although it is slightly more basic.

How Does It Work?

The Primal Diet involves the elimination of any processed foods and wheat and corn. Other foods to be avoided include all grains, soy, alcohol, refined oils, and the majority of sugars unless they are natural. Additionally, the consumption of raw dairy as a source of healthy fats is encouraged and guidelines suggest that any meat should be grass fed and both antibiotic and hormone free where possible. As the Primal Diet prioritises high quality, natural foods, it claims to improve your overall health and intake of nutrients, directly translating to weight loss through eating in a more natural way.

Who Is It For?

Almost everyone can benefit from following the primal diet as it relies on eating natural high-quality foods. It is claimed that some individuals may benefit more, including people with diabetes or food allergies, such as Celiac disease. It is a restrictive and sometimes inconvenient diet, so may not be suitable for everyone. As always, when eliminating any food group or type from your diet, it is recommended to consult with a health professional first.

★ **Find out More:**
The Primal Blueprint
By Mark Sisson

Great if....
*you love going
back to basics*

The Ration Diet

What is it?

The Ration Diet is a meal plan based on the recipes provided by the wartime Ministry of Food during World War II. It involves replacing modern day meals with those that are made from the allowed provisions. This diet is said to have multiple health and economic benefits that decrease your food bill, help you lose weight and encourage healthy eating habits.

How Does It Work?

The Ration Diet involves going back to basics and preparing a nutritious meal three times a day, making meals that include the provisions which were commonly allocated during the war. In general, a weekly adult ration allowed for 100g of Bacon and Ham, up to 226g of minced meat, 50g of butter, 50g of cheese, 100g of margarine, 100g of cooking fat, and three pints of milk. Additional rations were often provided less regularly, such as sugar and powdered eggs, and people were given a monthly points allowance with which they could buy foods in short supply. Families would also have bread, oats, fruit and vegetables. Due to the nature of rationing, lots of the recipes included vegetables, like leafy greens, cabbage, parsnip and potatoes. The Ration Diet is said to help you lose weight as you are avoiding processed foods and naturally decreasing your calorie intake through eating more nutrient-dense foods which fill you up, keep you satiated and prevent sugary cravings. Some followers of this diet also avoid using modern kitchen appliances, such as an electric whisk or toaster.

Who Is It For?

The Ration Diet appears to be suitable for the majority of people and does not target a specific group. It would not be suitable for vegetarians as the recipes include meat and some dairy. The diet involves considerable planning and preparation which can be time consuming and require some patience, so if you are looking for a diet which is quick and easy this meal plan may not be for you.

Great for....
portion control

★ **Find out More:**
The Ration Book Diet
By Mike Brown, Carol Harris & CJ Jackson

Raw Food Diet
Raw Foodism

What is it?

The Raw Food Diet is a lifestyle diet that promotes the eating of real foods in their natural state. Raw food is considered to be any food that has not been tinned, refined, processed or heated above 48C. This diet involves eating raw foods to obtain nutrients, without dangerous additives, in a manner that is easy to digest and that our bodies are naturally suited for. This diet is often mistaken for being the same, or similar, to the Primal and Paleo Diet, however with both of these other diets, cooked food is allowed.

How Does It Work?

The Raw Food Diet encourages eating unprocessed and uncooked foods. It is believed that the cooking of food destroys some of the food's natural enzymes, with this leading to the body overworking itself by producing more enzymes to digest the food and using up the energy in our bodies. Also, it is believed that cooking food above 57C destroys heat-sensitive nutrients, resulting in less nutrients being gained from the food. The eating of raw foods is said to increase energy levels, mental focus, overall health, and lead to stronger hair and nails.

There are several variations of the Raw Food Diet all with different rules and degrees to which foods can be cooked, with some including raw fish, raw dairy products (usually unpasteurised) and even some uncooked animal foods too. In the case of this diet, weight loss is not the main goal but you are likely to feel more full after eating lots of raw foods high in fibre and nutrients, this can curb cravings and result in eating less food overall.

Who Is It For?

The Raw Food Diet does not target one group of people. The main challenge for anyone on a Raw food diet is getting enough protein, vitamin B12 and iron as these are typically found in foods most of us prefer to cook such as meat, fish, eggs and grains.

★ **Find out More:**
The Raw Food Diet
By Christine Bailey

Great for....
cutting out cooking!

Rosemary Conley 3-2-1

What is it?

The Rosemary Conley 3-2-1 diet is an online subscription weight-loss service which provides eating plans that are designed to suit the way you eat and fit in with your lifestyle. It is claimed that there are three personality types which overweight people can be characterised in to: constant cravers, feasters and emotional eaters. The program shows you how to diet according to your personality type. The initial two phases involve a combination of 'light' and 'normal' eating days and are followed until you reach your target weight, with the final phase focusing on you staying slim - very much like the 5:2 Diet.

How Does It Work?

The 3-2-1 plan involves combining 'light' eating days where you consume 800 calorie and 'normal' eating days where you can eat and drink whatever you want, including treats high in fat. In the first week, it is recommended that you have 3 light eating days and 4 normal ones and in the next week you should have 2 light eating days and 5 normal days. The plan in the second week should be followed until you reach your weight loss goal. On reaching your target weight, in order to stay slim it is suggested that you follow the maintenance plan that involves restricting your calories for 1 day each week and having 6 normal eating days. Additionally, online followers have access to lots of recipes, how-to-cook video tutorials, a food and fitness diary, tools and motivation, all designed to help you lose weight and aid you to transition to a healthier lifestyle.

Who Is It For?

The 3-2-1 Diet appears suitable for most people and is aimed at individuals of all personality types who have found that calorie counting does not work for them. The program is simple, relatively easy to follow and not very restrictive. It has numerous recipes and meal plans to follow and caters for all dietary requirements, including having gluten and lactose free options.

Great for....
treat days

★ Find out More:
Rosemary Conley's 3-2-1 Diet
By Rosemary Conley

Sacred Heart Diet
The Vegetable Soup Diet

What is it?

The Sacred Heart Diet, also known as the 7-day Sacred Heart Diet or the Vegetable Soup Diet, is geared to help you quickly lose a lot of weight. It is claimed that you could lose between 10-17 pounds within 7 days. The diet was originally developed specifically for patients awaiting heart surgery who were required to lose weight quickly before their operation.

How Does It Work?

With the Sacred Heart Diet, a very strict plan must be followed and so a good level of discipline is required. Vegetable soup is a key component of the diet, a special recipe for the soup is provided and the dieter must have vegetable soup every single day. The dieter can have as much of the soup throughout the day as they like, but must have at least one portion at minimum. The rest of the strict food plan does allow the dieter some flexibility, providing a variety of limited, foods that they can choose from each day in addition to the vegetable soup. Although there are some alternatives that provide fish, this diet is really targeted for meat eaters with one day of the plan requiring between 10 and 20oz of beef. Due to the excessive and sporadic nature of this diet, it is highly recommended that you consult with a health professional first.

A list of 'allowed foods' is provided for each day; this list is very specific and quite limited, but is different for each of the seven days. Similar to elements of Weight Watchers and Slimming World, as long as the dieter selects from the specific list of allowed foods, the dieter can eat an unlimited amount of them.

Who Is It For?

This diet is great for you if you have good will power and can be very disciplined in controlling your intake. It is a quick fix; however it is not nutritionally balanced and so is not recommended for a long duration.

★ **Find out More:**
7 Day Sacred Heart Diet
By Gianna Rose

Great for....
quick fix weight loss

The Scarsdale Diet

What is it?

The Scarsdale Diet is a weight loss plan that offers a low carbohydrate, high protein and reduced fat approach, similar to other traditional diets. The difference with the Scarsdale Diet is that it consists of a two-week meal plan that should be strictly followed and claims to provide rapid weight loss.

How Does It Work?

The Scarsdale Diet involves eating exactly what is assigned and allows for the intake of lean meats, fresh fruit, and vegetables. It does not include any snacks between meals except carrot and broccoli. Due to the high level of protein intake appetite is suppressed and leaves you feeling fuller for longer. Additional guidelines include drinking at least four glasses of water a day, drinking both tea and coffee to increase metabolism, and walking 3km each day.

This diet is often followed by a Keep Trim Eating plan for another two weeks. This plan contains a higher number of calories and gives you more freedom by allowing the planning of your own menus, with a list of additional foods being permitted. It is suggested that these two plans should be continued in cycles until you reach your goal weight, with the Scarsdale Diet being intended for quick weight loss and not as a long-term lifestyle diet.

Who Is It For?

The Scarsdale Diet does not target one specific group of people, however it is quite a restrictive diet and requires willpower. The initial 2-week plan is very low in calories and you should consult with your GP before starting this diet, especially if pregnant or diagnosed with a medical condition.

Great for....
the disciplined dieter

★ **Find out More:**
The Complete Scarsdale Medical Diet
By Dr. Tarnowers

Sirtfood Diet

What is it?

The Sirtfood Diet is a two-phased approach that involves eating 'Sirtfoods" which are special foods that activate sirtuin proteins in the body. Sirtuins are thought to protect cells from dying when exposed to stress and are also believed to be involved in regulating inflammation, aging, and your body's ability to burn fat and maintain muscle by boosting your metabolism. This diet focuses on a lower calorie intake and sheds fat fast.

How Does It Work?

The Sirtfood Diet comprises two phases: the first phase lasts one week and involves restricting your calorie intake to 1000kcal per day for three days, with it being suggested that you have three sirtfood green juices and one meal rich in sirtfoods. The remaining four days involves increasing your calorie intake to 1500kcal by replacing one of the juices with another sirtfood-rich meal; such as chicken and kale curry or prawn stir-fry. The second phase of the Sirtfood Diet, also known as the maintenance phase, lasts 14 days in total and is claimed to be the phase in which steady weight loss occurs. Additionally, in the long-term the plan recommends eating three balanced meals rich in sirtfoods and one green juice daily.

Sirtfoods are said to be the best foods that nature has to offer with the most common sirtfoods including: dark chocolate (at least 85% cocoa); green tea, apples, citrus fruits, coffee, kale, blueberries and red wine. It is believed that by adding these healthy foods to your diet, effective and sustained weight loss occurs and improves your energy levels and overall health.

Who Is It For?

The Sirtfood Diet appears to be suitable for anybody, although it requires some willpower, as it can be difficult to maintain a 1000 calorie intake for three days. It is generally quite restrictive and requires planning and preparation but still allows for some treats.

★ **Find out More:**

The Sirtfood Diet
By Aidan Goggins and Glen Matten
The Sirt Diet Cookbook
By Jacqueline Whitehart

Great for....
chocolate & red wine lovers

SlimFast Diet

What is it?

SlimFast, like Weight Watchers and Slimming World, is a popular diet brand with a large following. SlimFast produce drink (shakes) and food products which act as complete meal and snack replacements. The diet is widely regarded as a quick fix weight loss although some people to follow the plan for an extended period of time.

How Does It Work?

Following a 3-2-1 concept, SlimFast dictates that the dieter controls their meals and snacks within the day. From a specific range, you can select 3 snacks, 2 meal replacements and 1 normal, well, balanced, meal. The snacks can be any fruit or vegetables, or alternatively any of the branded SlimFast snacks in their range. These can be bought online or at most major super markets.

Two of your three daily meals (most likely breakfast and lunch) must be a SlimFast meal replacement; this can be an actual Slim Fast meal or a SlimFast shake or bar. Your third meal of the day can be whatever you like, providing it is chosen from the select list of recipes, all of which are under 600 calories. The diet, obviously low in calories, is very structured but does provide a reasonable variety to choose from.

In addition to the 3-2-1 concept, SlimFast recommend that you also drink a minimum of 2 litres of water each day, and exercise alongside the diet.

Who Is It For?

SlimFast is great for busy people who have little time to prepare food. You eat three meals per day and three snacks per day, so it is great for those who like eating regularly and are self-confessed 'snackers'. Due to the low-calorie nature of the diet, it is recommended that you speak with your GP before beginning the Slim Fast Diet.

Great for....
snack lovers

★ **Find out More:**
SlimFast
slimfast.co.uk

Slimming World

What is it?

Slimming World is a monthly subscription service that provides food ideas centred on their diet plans. Support is provided through weekly meetings with other members and mentors, a lifestyle activity program, downloadable menus and recipes, and their own branded food range. Also, you can opt for an online-only membership, which provides a convenient 24/7 mode of support alongside all details of their Food Optimising Plan. Slimming World has a significant presence in the dieting world and has a very active members community.

How Does It Work?

By following the Slimming World Food Optimising Plan you have the freedom to create your own daily menus from a huge number of available recipes. They pride themselves on putting the individual in control of what they eat and not telling you what you can and can't eat, so you don't have to worry about counting points or weighing food. On the Food Optimising plan you are able to eat as much as you want, when you want, with no food types being banned.

The menus involve low-fat 'Free Foods' that can be eaten freely, such as fruit, veg, pasta, potatoes, lean meat and fish. The free foods are wholesome, filling, and healthy, leaving you satiated. Some foods are restricted, known as Syns, and should be enjoyed in moderation with a total number of Syns being allowed depending of your specific weight loss goals.

Who Is It For?

Slimming World seems to be suitable for anyone They provide a vast range of recipes that can cater for those with dietary requirements, as well as plans for breastfeeding women. The plan appears relatively easy to follow, allowing you to still enjoy the foods you love and instead of making you drastically change your lifestyle, you are encouraged to choose what works for you.

★ **Find out More:**

Slimming World
Slimmingworld.co.uk

Great for....
*freedom, flexibility
and support*

Slow Carb Diet
The 4 Hour Body Diet

What is it?

The Slow-Carb Diet involves sticking to an approved meal plan for 6 days a week with 1 cheat day being allowed, when you can eat whatever you want. The diet is based on the avoidance of foods that promote fat storage and it is claimed that you will rapidly burn fat, resulting in fast weight loss.

How Does It Work?

The Slow-Carb diet categorises foods into a number of main groups: animal protein, vegetables, legumes, spices, and oils and nuts. Typically, a slow-carb meal will be a combination of one food type from the first three groups and small amounts of the last. Generally, emphasis is placed on eating lean meats, beans and vegetables, whilst avoiding refined sugar, fruit, and white foods including bread, potatoes and pasta. You are allowed a cheat day each week, when you can eat any of the banned foods. The diet should boost your metabolism and help you lose excess fat with guidelines suggesting you should eat immediately after waking up, by starting your day with protein, and eating the same few meals over and over again.

Who Is It For?

The Slow-Carb diet appears to be suitable for anybody, however it is restrictive and repetitive, and so will require a lot of will power. As with most diets, you should consult with your GP before starting, especially if you are pregnant or suffering from a medical condition.

Great for....
fast results

★ Find out More:
The 4-Hour Body
Tim Ferriss

Smart Carb Diet
Super Carb Diet

What is it?

The Smart Carb Diet categorises carbohydrates as either 'good carbs' or 'bad carbs'. It seeks to eliminate bad carbs from your eating habits; which includes some of our modern days staples such as white bread, white rice and potatoes. Instead it encourages good carbs such as grainy bread, brown rice legumes and starchy vegetables. The diet is sometimes calorie counted, although not always, and usually has an initial time plan attached to it (for example 5 weeks) after which you should see results.

How Does It Work?

Bad carbs are basically refined foods that are quickly digested and absorbed into the body. They enter the bloodstream rapidly causing blood sugar levels to spike which in turn triggers a surge of insulin.

Insulin is an important hormone which signals cells in your muscles to absorb the sugar and power them with fuel. Insulin then directs any unused sugar into storage - in your fat cells. The end result of this is you eat more than you need to, but you don't feel satisfied so you're looking around for a snack an hour later.

If however you replace these carbohydrates with good carbs they are digested less quickly and don't create the sugar spike. These good carbs should therefore help you feel fuller BEFORE you've overeaten and 'stick with you' for longer after a meal.

Who Is It For?

This diet is good for anyone who wants to lose weight and eat well by cutting out highly processed food from their diet. It is a slow & steady approach that can provide long lasting, if not dramatic, results.

★ **Find out More:**

Davina's Smart Carbs
By Davina McCall

Great if....
*if you feel hungry
most of the time*

Smart For Life

What is it?

Smart For Life is a weight management program that provides meal replacements designed to control hunger and provide you with the highest amounts of nutrition. Their products are made with natural ingredients and are scientifically formulated to be an ideal balance of fibre, protein and complex carbs that naturally suppress appetite.

How Does It Work?

Smart For Life diet is based on the idea that your body can only shed fat under certain conditions, with the program claiming to create these necessary conditions, such as a correct protein to sugar ratio in the food you eat, a low Glycaemic Index and Glycaemic Load.

The guidelines for weight loss include eating one cookie every two to three hours, six times a day or by eating the equivalent in protein bars, shakes or soups, followed by a dinner consisting of lean protein and green, leafy vegetables. The Smart For Life Store provides you with the products containing the necessary nutrients at a cost and you only have to prepare one meal a day yourself. There is also online support and weight loss kits available online to aid you in the program. Overall, the program is designed to aid in weight loss, increase energy, reduce inflammation and improve sleep through consuming clean foods multiple times a day.

Who Is It For?

The Smart For Life program appears to be for anyone, although the majority of meal replacements contain egg or milk and so it would be difficult to follow if you have specific dietary requirements. The program requires little preparation or effort but may be difficult to follow as it is quite restrictive and repetitive in what you can eat.

Great for....
convenient meal replacements

★ **Find out More:**
Smart for Life
Smartforlife.com

The Smoothie Diet

What is it?

The Smoothie Diet is a low-calorie plan that involves drinking smoothies to lose weight, tone up or just stay healthy. There are various Smoothie diets that you can follow with numerous customisable recipes that can be adapted to help you reach weight loss or health goals. The use of smoothies is advocated as they help you lose weight by getting all the necessary nutrients in one glass without adding any excess or empty calories. In many aspects, this is quite similar to the Liquid Diet.

How Does It Work?

Smoothies are a convenient and healthy way to diet and should contain a good balance of protein, healthy fats and complex carbohydrates as well as vitamins and minerals. The plan generally restricts your calorie intake over a certain period of time, for example 7 days, replacing your meals with smoothies to aid fast weight loss and detoxify the body.

The diet involves smoothies which contain lots of green vegetables and low-calorie, low-sugar fruits, such as berries. Leafy greens make up a large part of smoothies as they contain fibre and can bulk up a smoothie without adding many calories. Additionally, protein should be added to your smoothies as proteins curb hunger and aid weight loss. Protein powders, such as whey, soy or casein can be used although protein can be added without the use of supplements, for example by adding silken tofu or Greek yoghurt. The diet also allows for low-calorie natural flavourings to be added such as cocoa powder or cinnamon which can help prevent boredom. Foods to avoid include canned fruits or vegetables, full fat dairy, fruit juice and fruit high in sugar.

Who Is It For?

The Smoothie Diet appears to be suitable for everyone, there are thousands of smoothie recipes to follow although some can be more calorific than you might imagine, so be selective. Low-calorie, restrictive diets can be hard to stick to. They require will power and a certain degree of planning and preparation. It is advised that you consult with your GP before starting any diet.

★ Find out More:

500 Juices and Smoothies
By Christine Watson
The Smoothie Recipe Book
By Mendocino Press

Great for....
smoothies lovers

The Sonoma Diet

What is it?

The Sonoma Diet is influenced by a Mediterranean plant-focused way of eating and places emphasis on nutrient dense foods. Its creator claims that besides losing weight, the plan will help you break your sugar addiction and teach you to satisfy cravings with healthy foods. It is a simple approach that contains some elements of the raw food diet and primal diet, with a little bit more flexibility.

How Does It Work?

The Sonoma Diet consists of three waves in total and although there is no formal exercise component followers are encouraged to engage in daily activity. Additionally, the diet controls portion size by specifying the plate to bowl size for breakfast and dinner. The first wave is 10 days long and is designed to promote quick weight loss. In this wave followers are encouraged to eliminate processed foods, natural sugars and some vegetables, and are allowed to consume lean beef, eggs, and some oils. The main emphasis is on high-nutrient foods, including almonds, broccoli, strawberries, spinach and whole grains. The second wave gives you slightly more flexibility and allows you to add in some fruits, more vegetables, some wine and sugar-free treats. Guidelines suggest that dieters only move into the third wave once their ideal weight has been reached. The third wave focuses on making the Sonoma Diet a part of your lifestyle, not just a one-off diet fix, and encourages experimenting with different fruits, enjoying rare treats and having fun with fitness.

Who Is It For?

The Sonoma Diet appears to be for anybody and has various meal plans, recipes and smart food combinations that you can use. It also caters for dietary restrictions or preferences, allowing meat-free protein sources like soy and eggs, as long as they are low in saturated fat. The first wave is fairly restrictive but the last two are well balanced, so if you are able to complete the first phase it does become easier and more flexible.

Great for....
rapid lasting weight loss

★ Find out More:
The Sonoma Diet
By Connie Guttersen

Soup Diet

What is it?

A Soup Diet is often a 7-day plan that involves eating as much as you like of a low calorie soup alongside a specific meal plan of different food combinations, with soup replacing one or more of your daily meals. The Soup Diet claims to provide you with the nutrients you need and helps you burn fat. The diet is specifically geared for rapid weight loss. It is very similar to the Smoothie Diets and the Liquid Diet, but provides a wider variety of options.

How Does It Work?

A Soup Diet claims to clean your body of impurities, provide you with more energy and a sense of well-being whilst rapidly burning fat, resulting in weight loss. Low calorie soups are said to be great for weight loss as they are more filling per calorie due to their high water content and high amount of fibre, this leads to a decrease in appetite and cravings. Additionally, a bowl of soup can help warm you up by increasing your core temperature leading to a boost in metabolism and your circulation; this results in fat burn and also a natural cleanse of toxins in your body. Generally, the soups are packed with vegetables, protein and complex carbohydrates, with the best soups containing carrots, onions, cabbage, or celery. Soup Diets also recommend avoiding alcohol, sweets and wheat. You are encouraged to incorporate regular exercise into your lifestyle and to hydrate regularly, with water, tea, 100% fruit juice or black coffee.

Who Is It For?

A Soup Diet is specifically targeted at those who want to lose weight quickly. Often a precise plan is followed; so little planning is required although the preparation can be time consuming at first. This diet provides a wide variety of soup recipes and is suitable for those with dietary requirements as the majority are vegetable based. It is advised that you consult with your GP before starting a soup-based diet and it is not recommended for those who are pregnant or breastfeeding.

★ **Find out More:**
The Big Healthy Soup Diet
By Linda Lazarides

Great for....
the winter months

The South Beach Diet

What is it?

The South Beach Diet is a simple eating plan developed by Florida based Cardiologist Dr. Agatston. It concentrates on eating high-fibre, low-glycaemic carbohydrates, unsaturated fats, and lean protein.

How Does It Work?

The diet is split into three phases. In phase One (which lasts for 14 days) most carbohydrates are banned to give the body a complete rest from fluctuating blood sugar and insulin levels. Foods that are not allowed include bread, rice, potatoes, pasta, fruit, milk, sweets, cake, biscuits, ice cream, sugar and alcohol. The focus is on eating lean meat, chicken, fish, eggs, low-fat cheese, some nuts and olive oil.

In Phase Two, low GI carbs including most fruits, granary bread, wholegrain cereals, pasta and low-fat milk are reintroduced. This phase is continued until you reach your target weight.

Phase Three sees the introduction of an even wider variety of foods and is how you keep your weight steady for the rest of your life.

For each phase, there are no limits on portion sizes - you simply eat enough to satisfy your appetite - and you're encouraged to eat three meals and snacks each day.

Who Is It For?

This diet is for people who want to see reasonably fast results and with the intention of making a lifelong lifestyle change.

Great for....
shifting stubborn belly fat

★ Find out More:
The South Beach Diet Plan
By Dr Arthur Agatston

The Sugar Detox

What is it?

The Sugar Detox aims to break the addictive cycle of sugar, with its feel good highs and crashes, in as little as three days. The detox claims that sugar addictions are making us fat, sick and causing premature aging, so eliminating sugar can reverse these damages and lead to weight loss and an overall improvement in health. As with many detox plans, this is great for quick weight loss.

How Does It Work?

The sugar detox initially involves a three-day detox where all sugars are eliminated. This includes carbohydrates like wheat, grains, alcohol, food with added sugar, in addition to the avoidance of fruit and dairy products. You are allowed to eat whole sources of protein, plenty of vegetables, and healthy fat sources. After completing the three-day detox, you can gradually reintroduce healthy sugars, starting with an apple and a serving of dairy each day. Following this more fruit, grains and dairy can be added into your diet and there is a recommended 4-week eating plan to follow that provides meal plans and recipes to help dieters maintain a low sugar diet.

Additionally, there are several different sugar detoxes available all with a varying amount of time spent without sugar, and all allowing slightly different foods to be reintroduced.

Who Is It For?

The Sugar Detox seems to be specific for those who want to lose weight, feel they consume too much sugar, or experience an addictive sugar cycle. It is advised to consult with your GP before starting this diet, and several side effects have been commonly noted during the detox, including headaches and crankiness. This detox is great for those wanting to shift pounds fast.

★ Find out More:

The Sugar Detox
By Brooke Alpert
Sugar Detox for Beginners
By Hayward Press

Great for....
*breaking that
addictive sweet cycle*

Sugar-Free Diet

What is it?

A Sugar-Free Diet is a lifestyle change that typically limits all sources of food with added sugar and hidden sugar. Often, it is encouraged to also reduce your intake of high carbohydrate foods, such as grains, and fruits as they contain natural sugars. This diet is based on the idea that the removal of excess sugar from your diet not only aids weight loss but also can reduce your risk of common health issues, including digestive problems and type 2 diabetes. This is very similar to the Sugar Detox, but with more of a long-term approach.

How Does It Work?

Sugar Free diets can vary in the types of sugar they allow you to eat. Generally, dieters are encouraged to eat balanced meals consisting of proteins, plenty of vegetables, healthy fats, nuts and seeds, all of which are nutrient dense and are designed to replace the "empty" calories of foods high in sugar. Processed food and drinks high in sugar should be avoided, including alcohol and artificially sweetened drinks.

Most of the low sugar or sugar free diet plans do not require you to count calories or weigh foods as the elimination of processed and high sugar foods is usually enough to produce weight loss on its own. Additionally, it is claimed that Sugar Free diets help balance your blood sugar levels throughout the day, prevent you from developing some diseases, control your appetite and keep you fuller and energised for longer.

Who Is It For?

The Sugar Free diet does not appear to target a specific group of people, and there are a variety of different plans available depending on your goal and dietary requirements or preferences. It may be slightly inconvenient to follow due to having to plan and prepare your own meals. This diet is for those looking for a long-term new approach to food and diet, rather than a quick fix.

Great for....
those in it for the long run

★ **Find out More:**
Sugar-Free Diet Plan
By Dr. Axe

Vegan Diet

What is it?

Veganism is not just about food it is a lifestyle choice. Vegans attempt to exclude all forms of animal exploitation from their lives whether for food, clothing or any other purpose. As such a vegan diet does not contain any animal products at all; this includes meat, eggs and dairy.

How Does It Work?

Whilst there is no defined plan for a general vegan diet, there are lots of variants of veganism including :

Whole-food vegan diet: Includes whole plant foods such as fruits, vegetables, whole grains, legumes, nuts and seeds.

Raw-food vegan diet: Includes raw fruits, vegetables, nuts, seeds.

Fruitarian Diet: A raw-food vegan diet that limits fat-rich plants.

The Starch Solution: A low-fat, high-carb vegan diet that focuses on cooked starches like potatoes, rice and corn instead of fruit.

Raw till 4: A diet which allows only raw foods to be consumed until 4 p.m., with the option of a cooked plant-based meal for dinner.

A vegan diet usually has an emphasis on nutritious, whole plant foods and, as there is a limit to the amount of processed food eaten, this may help you lose weight. Studies have shown that those adopting a vegan diet tend to be thinner and have a lower body mass index (BMI). However as veganism is usually a lifestyle choice this weight loss may in part be explained by factors other than diet: including physical activity and other health-related behaviours.

Who Is It For?

Veganism is a great way to change the way you look at food and make a positive impact on the world and animal welfare. It may not provide dramatic results fast but, if properly balanced with supplements, a vegan diet can make you healthier and leaner.

★ **Find out More:**

The New Vegan
By Aine Carlin
Vegan Cookbook for Beginners
By Rockridge Press

Great for....
making a
positive life change

Vegetarian Diet

What is it?

Generally speaking a vegetarian is someone who doesn't eat meat. However that definition is too simple as there are several variations of a vegetarian diet. The traditional vegetarian is Lacto-ovo which means they eat eggs and dairy but do not eat fish, meat or any other animal product that has been produced as a result of the animal's death. Other variations include lacto vegetarian, ovo vegetarian and of course Vegan.

How Does It Work?

Vegetarians are typically leaner than meat eaters as a vegetarian diet usually contains less saturated fat and focuses on foods such as fruits, vegetables and whole grains which often have less calories than a traditional diet. Vegetarian diets however are not automatically low calorie and do not always lead to weight loss. Counting calories and keeping track of portion sizes at each meal is still required as with any conventional diet. Whole, unprocessed foods and the reduction of processed sugars are the best choices.

Who Is It For?

Vegetarianism is a good way to change your eating habits and make a positive impact on the world and animal welfare. It may not provide dramatic results quickly but a healthy vegetarian diet can make you healthier and leaner.

Great for....
the environment

★ **Find out More:**
The Hairy Dieters Go Veggie
By Hairy Bikers
The Skinny Vegetarian Slow Cooker Book
By CookNation

Very Low Calorie Diet
VLCD Liquid Diet

What is it?

A very low calorie diet is an eating plan that includes very low (sometimes extremely low) daily food consumption. It is defined as a diet of 800 calories a day (often less) which are usually consumed as liquid meals. The liquid meal replacements contain the recommended daily requirements of vitamins, minerals, trace elements, fatty acids and protein, with carbs entirely absent or substituted for a portion of protein.

How Does It Work?

The liquid products associated with the VLCD diet are usually sold as a powder that are mixed with water or another low-food-energy liquid. The diet should only be undertaken with medical supervision and should be followed for a maximum of 12 weeks.

Who Is It For?

A VLCD is only usually suitable for an obese person who needs to lose a lot of weight quickly. This diet can present a risk to health and is only usually recommended when the health risk of obesity is considered much greater than any risks of the diet itself.

Great if....
you are obese,
and want
to make a change fast

★ Find out More:
Total Solution Diet Plan
exantediet.com

The Virgin Diet

What is it?

The Virgin Diet is an online subscription weight loss program that claims to help you hit your weight loss goals more easily and faster with a plan that is specific to your needs. The plan advocates removing foods that can be offensive to your body, with this providing a number of health benefits such as better sleep, increased energy and weight loss.

How Does It Work?

The Virgin Diet lasts for 3-weeks and is based on the idea that people are unable to tolerate certain foods and this can result in inflammation, weight gain, skin issues and other health problems. The plan encourages eliminating gluten, dairy, soy, eggs, peanuts and sugar, and emphasises eating fruit, vegetables, protein, healthy fats and gluten-free grains. After 3-weeks followers should reintroduce the foods one-by-one and monitor their symptoms. Any foods that they cannot tolerate are then eliminated for good. The diet claims that through fighting food intolerances and eating plenty of anti-inflammatory foods, this will boost your metabolism and help you feel less bloated and healthier. The online subscription also provides meal-by-meal support, lots of recipes and a fitness program, all designed to help you to reach your weight loss goal.

Who Is It For?

The Virgin Diet is targeted at individuals who are resistant to weight loss or who suffer from food sensitivities and intolerances, however it appears to be suitable for everyone. The diet is restrictive and requires time and patience when going through the cycles of reintroduction. It is advised that you consult with a medical professional before starting this diet.

Great for....
food intolerance

★ Find out More:
IThe Virgin Diet
By JJ Virgin

Weight Watchers

What is it?

Weight Watchers has a very large presence in the dieting world. It is a monthly subscription service which provides ideas and support around their diet plans. There are local weekly meetings you can attend supported by mentors and other members, recipes to download, and their own branded meals and snacks are available in most supermarkets.

How Does It Work?

There are two different approaches with Weight Watchers. The first option is a plan where a number of points are allocated to each item of food and drink, and you must stick to a set number of points in a day; providing you do not exceed the number of points, you can eat whatever you like! The other is a 'no count' plan where rather than counting points for every item of food, a list of foods that you can eat is provided instead. If there are some foods that you just cannot survive without, and these are not on the list, you still have a small selection of points to use how you please for little extra treats.

Who Is It For?

Weight Watchers appears to be suitable for anybody - there is no specific criteria and the plan is not targeted at any specific groups. They provide a wide range of recipes including a vegetarian and gluten-free range for those with dietary requirements. Almost all meals include preparing the meal from scratch, so a certain amount of organisation is required to begin with - although a range of pre-made supermarket meals does exist.

★ **Find out More:**
Weight Watchers
weightwatchers.co.uk

Great if....
*you want to keep eating
the foods you love*

Wheat Belly Diet

What is it?

The Wheat Belly Diet is an online subscription plan based on the idea that eliminating wheat from our diets is a 'path to health' that can result in several health benefits, with one of these being weight loss. The plan claims that it is more of a lifestyle diet as opposed to one that restricts calories or involves excessive exercise. The Wheat Belly Diet is similar to the Gluten Free Diet through the concept of eliminating grains.

How Does It Work?

The Wheat Belly diet is mainly based on two principles: eliminating wheat and other gluten-containing grains, such as rye and barley; and managing carbohydrate levels to help lower your blood sugar levels and promote weight loss. Essentially, all wheat products are removed as foods containing wheat flour cause your blood sugar levels to elevate much higher and more quickly than most other foods.

Additionally, wheat is said to contain compounds that stimulate your appetite and cause overeating, this results in the build up of fats around your abdomen, known as "Wheat Belly". In eliminating wheat, this helps you to satisfy your appetite, keep you feeling fuller for longer, and curb your cravings. The diet provides you with meal plans and several recipes to follow, with ingredients including 'real' and natural foods such as fish, meat, nuts, eggs, olives, oils, and almond flour instead of wheat-containing flour.

Who Is It For?

The Wheat Belly Diet appears to be suitable for everybody, with numerous recipes being available and several dietary requirements being catered for. This diet, in certain variations, may be great for those with gluten intolerances. It is advised that you should consult with your GP before beginning this diet, especially if you are taking medication, are unwell, pregnant or breast-feeding.

Great for....
getting rid of that bloated feeling

* Find out More:
Wheat Belly
By Dr. William Davis

The Whole Foods Diet

What is it?

Following a Whole Food Diet means cutting all processed foods out of your diet and maximizing your nutrient intake from natural sources such as vegetables, fruits, nuts, organic eggs, meat, fish & poultry. It is not designed as a weight loss diet although steady weight loss can be a happy side effect of switching to a Whole Foods Diet. Some plans encourage a month long period of introduction to convince you of the positive effects. There is also a plant-based version of this diet that cuts out all the animal products.

How Does It Work?

A Whole Food Diet is based around the belief that eating more whole foods is the best way to improve health and prevent disease. Whole foods retain their fibre, phytochemicals and the nutrients that are often removed in processed foods. The Whole Food movement was born in the 1980's 'to provide a more natural alternative to what the food supply was typically offering at the time'.

When you eat whole foods, you are eating food in its most nutritious form. If it grows in the ground or is farmed/fished/hunted, you can eat it. Things that cannot be eaten are junk/processed food. Whole food is basically fresh produce of any kind: fresh vegetables, fresh (and dried) fruit, dairy products without added sugar or chemical flavourings and fresh unprocessed meat, poultry, and fish. Legumes and nuts are also good along with any products made from them - as long as they are made without added sugar, unhealthy fats, or chemicals.

Who Is It For?

A Whole Food diet is recommended for people who wish to monitor the type of food they are eating and the way in which it is produced. It is essentially a return to 'real' food. The health effects are lasting and gradual weight loss is a natural effect of cutting processed food out of your diet.

★ **Find out More:**
The 30 Day Whole Food Challenge
By Emily Willis

Great for....
fans of simple healthy food

Zero Belly Diet

What is it?

The Zero Belly Diet is a program featuring week-by-week meal plans that are designed for those who struggle to lose weight, particularly from around the belly area. It is claimed that the diet shows you how to deactivate fat genes, increase your metabolism and restore a healthy digestive balance, all without having to count calories or spend several hours a day at the gym.

How Does It Work?

The Zero Belly Diet recommends starting with a cleanse in order to lose weight quickly while avoiding the pitfall of yo-yo dieting. This is implemented using a 7-day meal plan that reduces your calorie intake a little, without drastically altering the way in which you eat and it also includes short bursts of mild exercise to increase your metabolism. The Zero Belly Diet claims to keep your body fuelled using high-nutrient, clean foods that improve your health and target your belly fat on a genetic level. There are several recipes to follow for meals, snacks and desserts, all of which are balanced to get rid of belly fat.

Who Is It For?

The Zero Belly Diet appears to be for everyone, especially those who struggle with getting rid of excess fat around the stomach. As there are many recipes, this diet is easy to follow and can be adapted for used for those with special dietary requirements. Long lasting results can be achieved.

Great for....
blasting unwanted belly fat

★ **Find out More:**
Zero Belly Diet
By David Zinczenko

The Zone Diet

What is it?

The Zone Diet is focused on low carbohydrate intake, but was specifically developed in order to reduce inflammation induced by diet. It claims to aid weight loss, reduce the risk of chronic disease and improve overall performance as part of a life-long dietary program. The Zone is an optimal bodily state and it is believed that the secret to maintaining wellness is being in the 'Zone'.

How Does It Work?

In this diet the 'Zone' is described as a physiological state in your body and if you are in the 'Zone' you have optimised your ability to control diet-induced inflammation. The inflammation is said to be the reason that you become sick, gain weight, and age faster. Overall, there are 3 clinical markers that define if you are in the 'Zone' with all three ideal values having to be met. These markers can be measured using blood work, cellular inflammation tests and blood sugar levels, aided by your doctor.

The Zone diet requires that you eat a balanced meal consisting of: protein such as fish, egg whites or lean beef making up 1/3 of your plate and being the size of your palm, carbohydrates making up 2/3 of your plate, such as colourful vegetables and fruit, avoiding those high in sugar or starch; and a little monounsaturated fat is allowed, such as avocado or olive oil. The guidelines recommend eating three meals a day and two snacks to prevent overeating; ensuring grains and starches are restricted to reach an optimal level of protein to glycaemic load. In addition to the diet plan it is also suggested that dieters take anti-inflammatory supplements and purified polyphenol supplements in order to stay in the 'Zone' and reduce inflammation.

Who Is It For?

The Zone Diet does not specifically target one group of people, although it does stress the anti-inflammatory benefits. However, it is advised you consult with you GP before starting the diet as a treatment for inflammatory disease. This diet is great for those looking to eat many of the foods they love without eliminating too many foods, and allows you to easily control portion size without having to count calories.

★ **Find out More:**
The Zone Diet
By Barry Sears

Great for....
reducing inflammation